THE VERY BEST
PAINKILLER
FOODS

5/14

Rachel Fontaine

THE VERY BEST
PAINKILLER
FOODS

72 Natural Foods to Ease
Arthritis and Joint Pain

115 Healing Recipes

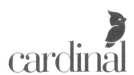

cardinal

Rachel Fontaine

The Very Best Painkiller Foods
Superfoods to Ease Arthritis and Joint Pain
115 Healing Recipes

Graphic design: Luc Sauvé
Layout for English version: Richard Morrissette
English translation: Joëlle Bernier
Copyediting: Martine Gagnon

Recipe photography: pages 41 (persimmon), 84, 91 (sesame seeds), 92, 95, 96, 98, 99, 100, 102, 105, 109 (celery seeds) 114, 115, 116, 117, 127, 139, 155, 173, 187, 203, 217, 231, 243 and 255 by Claude Charlebois with Linda McKenty, Food Stylist. All other photographs (except cover) by Julie Léger.

Cover photography: Tango
Food stylist: Véronique Gagnon-Lalanne
Cover design: natalicommunication design

We acknowledge the financial support of the Government of Canada through the Book Publishing Industry Development Program (BPIDP) for our publishing activities and the support of the Government of Quebec through the tax credits for book publishing program – SODEC.

ISBN: 978-2-920943-75-9

Legal Deposit – Library and Archives Canada, 2014
              Bibliothèque et Archives Nationales du Québec, 2014

Printed in Canada

Eating for pleasure

Without a doubt, eating is one of life's greatest pleasures. My partner of thirty years and I both believe that eating goes beyond sustenance. Over the years, we have grown to enjoy preparing our food together; we then enjoy sharing the fruits of our labor. Our culinary experiences have taken shape over the course of our travels through many countries and we now take great pleasure in cooking foods influenced by many different cuisines.

Lately though, our eating habits have changed. Our respective jobs have led us to take an interest in nutrition and the role of food in health. Personally, three years of research and preparation for my first book on the benefits of certain foods, has had a ripple effect. Through my reading, I discovered that many fruits and vegetables have the power to relieve joint pain, particularly osteoarthritis pain, which has afflicted me for the past ten years. When put to the test, the information I had gathered, combined with gradual diet changes that put more emphasis on foods with anti-inflammatory properties known to mankind for centuries, I was able to diminish wear and tear on my joints. Without becoming vegetarian per say, I reduced meat consumption by a third, eliminated most processed foods from my diet, cut down on fat and sugar and, especially, started eating raw vegetables.

In fact, serendipity led me to rediscover the pleasure of eating raw foods. My spouse and I were on vacation and had stopped along the way to try out the area's best restaurant. It was August, at the peak of tourist season. The restaurant was full and service slow; it was almost an hour before we were served. A basketful of freshly-picked vegetables adorned each table, evidently in order to appease hungry patrons. I appreciated the intention, but thought the effort lacking for such an establishment - entire vegetables devoid of the simplest preparation. Ripe tomatoes, scrubbed carrots, a sweet pepper, a few beans with no garnish other than their shiny skin and bright color. But we were so hungry that we dove in, munching the tomatoes like apples, savoring the sweetness and crunch of the carrots, pepper and beans. I don't remember what we ate after that except that it was as good as we had expected. The most vivid memory of that meal is the unusual appetizer that brought me back to my childhood when, for a few short summery weeks, my mother would serve us produce from her tiny, but lovingly-tended, garden.

It would be a lie to say that ever since then I have been eating more vegetables. It took a few more months and a few coincidences – such as research for the book I was about to write – before I decided to reintroduce crudités to the menu. In the pile of books I had to research in order to write a book on the subject of health, I discovered that a number of fruits and vegetables have anti-inflammatory properties and contain antioxidants that attack oxygen-derived free radicals, which are harmful, particularly to joints. I had osteoarthritis and the doctor had warned me: back and hip pain following a pelvic fracture would only worsen with age.

He half-heartedly suggested I consult a physiotherapist who then designed an exercise program for me to follow. I owe her a certain degree of pain-relief and benefit from a ten-minute workout session that I still do religiously twice a day. But I also would not go without the foods that have now become part of my daily diet: before my evening meal I start with a simple first course of greens – arugula, spinach or endive – with pepper and zucchini slices, broccoli and cauliflower florets, melon and pineapple cubes and, when in season, slices of ripe tomato and cucumber. And even though I believe this plate full of color is responsible for alleviating some of my pain, it is the taste that I enjoy the most. I am not alone--my feasting companion has also taken to enjoying the taste and the benefits of this dietary ritual. We are close in age, and he had also started to feel pain in his hands and knees.

We were accustomed to rich and varied foods, but it is with loyal enthusiasm that we continue to benefit from this daily crudité regimen that, without being miraculous, allows us to lead healthier lives. We wrote this book together. Denis did the research and contributed to writing the first part; he also collaborated closely on the recipe section, tasting and critiquing each of the 115 recipes that I created and reinvented. All of these were prepared with a focus on foods that help relieve joint pain. Although most of the recipes avoid red meat and dairy products, such as butter, cream and milk, you will find that they are not exclusively vegetarian. There is a chapter devoted to poultry and rabbit that will satisfy carnivorous appetites. The foods that I suggest are not restrictive or bland; on the contrary, my goal in writing this book has always been to promote tasty foods that are beneficial to people suffering from joint pain, while avoiding foods that are harmful. The foods we recommend are not part of a strict diet and are therefore enjoyable to all, whether or not you suffer from joint pain. We hope you enjoy these foods as much as we do, and feel the benefits they have to offer on a daily basis!

Part One

Diet and Arthritis

If you are reading this book then you or a loved one most likely suffers from arthritis. You hope to find a way to improve your health and alleviate your pain. You are looking to nutrition to accomplish this and rightly so. The foods we eat play an important role in all diseases, including arthritis. Before we examine the role of foods and those that can be beneficial, let's look at the different types of arthritis. Arthritis encompasses at least one hundred joint inflammation disorders. Not so long ago these were called rheumatism, and even today, the specialists that treat them are called rheumatologists.

Which one do you suffer from?

The two most frequent joint diseases are osteoarthritis and rheumatoid arthritis. The other most common types of arthritis – less frequent but still affecting a large number of people – are gout, systemic lupus erythematosus (SLE) and ankylosing spondylitis.

If you suffer from osteoarthritis or rheumatoid arthritis, you are not alone. Osteoarthritis (OA), also known as degenerative joint disease, is the most common form of arthritis. Overall OA affects 13.9% of adults aged 25 and older and 33.6% (12.4 million) of those 65+ totaling an estimated 26.9 million US adults in 2005 – up from 21 million in 1990 (believed to be conservative estimate).

Do you know which type of arthritis you suffer from? Many people have aches and pains in their joints and bones, blaming their rheumatism without knowing what their condition really is. Similar symptoms and ambiguous terminology add to the confusion. Is it inflammation, infection, swelling or joint dysfunction? For health professionals, including nutritionists, is it important to determine the nature of the disorder in order to prescribe correct treatment and diet to reduce pain and slow down the disease.

If you are not sure of the type of arthritis or rheumatism you suffer from, see your doctor and try and get an exact diagnosis. You can also consult the American Arthritis Society to help identify your condition.

Osteoarthritis: Osteoarthritis is a disease characterized by degeneration of cartilage and its underlying bone within a joint, as well as bony overgrowth. The breakdown of these tissues eventually leads to pain and joint stiffness. The joints most commonly affected are the knees, hips, and those in the hands and spine. The specific causes of osteoarthritis are unknown, but are believed to be a result of both mechanical and molecular events in the affected joint. Disease onset is gradual and usually begins after the age of 40.

Rheumatoid arthritis: Rheumatoid arthritis is a systemic inflammatory disease which manifests itself in multiple joints of the body. The inflammatory process primarily affects the lining of the joints (synovial membrane), but can also affect other organs such as the heart and lungs. The inflamed synovium leads to erosions of the cartilage and bone and sometimes joint deformity. Pain, swelling, and redness are common joint complaints.

Osteoarthritis usually affects the hands, feet, knees, backbone and hips, while rheumatoid arthritis mostly affects hand and foot joints.

If gout is your problem, it is of utmost importance that it be properly diagnosed. Gout is a rheumatic disease resulting from the deposition of uric acid crystals (monosodium urate) in tissues and fluids within the body. This process is caused by an overproduction or under excretion of uric acid. Certain common medications, alcohol, and foods are known to be contributory factors.

Acute gout will typically manifest itself as an acutely red, hot, and swollen joint with excruciating pain. Some of the foods to be avoided are: sardines, mackerel, herring, peas, spinach and tea (even though these are thought to relieve some types of arthritis). Other foods to be avoided are: liver, seafood, sweetbreads, deli meats, beer and coffee.

Do you know what you are eating?

If one is to examine arthritis from a nutritional point of view, one has to consider the complex nature of the foods we eat. This aspect has long impeded scientists and health professionals from making connections between food and arthritis. The medical community is still skeptical on this issue even after establishing direct correlations in certain conditions such as gout and even after many studies over recent years have confirmed the hypothesis - previously considered silly or reserved for alternative medicine - that there are good and bad foods.

But the problem is that we do not eat singular foods, and we rarely consume them in their natural form. Truth is we don't really know what we are eating. The typical North-American diet is composed mostly of extensively transformed foods loaded with chemicals. Hundreds of food additives are authorized: coloring agents, preservatives, emulsifiers, thickeners, gelling ingredients, artificial flavoring, acidulants, acidity regulators, anti-caking compounds, processing salt, firmness agents, sweeteners--they are all part of our diet, whether we are aware of them or not.

It is practically impossible to know exactly what is in processed foods. Are the ingredients listed on the label really as harmless as claimed by health agencies? They may be safe in the short-term but what about long-term? How are we to know if what we are eating is good or bad for our health, and if it has an effect on disease?

Moreover, we eat while simultaneously taking medication and supplements. All these things mix and blend in our bodies for better or for worse.

Fortunately, more and more studies are on the same wavelength, confirming that, yes, there is a link between diet, health and disease; yes, some foods are bad for us, full of fat, salt and sugar; yes, some foods are good for us, when consumed fresh, with as little transformation as possible, allowing them to prevent disease and alleviate symptoms, and even, hypothetically, perhaps even cure some diseases.

Taking stock

To what degree can you blame your diet for your health problems, particularly your arthritis? How can you make positive changes to your eating habits? No doctor, nutritionist or specialist can say. It is all on you.

I urge you to keep reading and take stock of what you consume in order to find a way to make certain changes without sacrificing the pleasures of eating. This is the goal of this book: to help people with arthritis fight their condition, improve their health, and prevent other diseases, all the while enjoying nutritious and tasty meals and discovering new foods.

Diet: the first step in any treatment

First, a word of caution. Diet is only one component of any disease treatment. Even though the foods we eat are among the usual suspects for many modern conditions and diseases such as obesity, cardiovascular disease and cancer, they do not cause disease directly, any more or less than being the only remedy for disease. Traditional treatments, medications, supplements (such as glucosamine), physical activity, the environment, alternative medicine thought to have an effect on joint disease (hydrotherapy, massotherapy, relaxation, yoga, etc.), all have a role to play in fighting disease. Only in conjunction with the above, can an appropriate diet show good results.

That said, I firmly believe that a healthy diet is the basis for any treatment, simply because we have to eat to live. We ate before getting sick and before feeling joint pain. We continue eating despite chronic disease and despite the evolution of our state of health. The diet that provides essential nutrients each day for our survival is affected by our actual nutritional needs, as well as by our moods and tastes.

When we are sick, we have to give our body the best possible nutrients to fight disease, whether by eating foods that build resistance, that counteract medication side-effects or that help heal invasive surgery.

A healthy diet has many important roles to play:

- Ensuring best over-all health
- Fighting pain
- Slowing disease progression
- Preventing disease onset

Weight control: a key factor in treating arthritis

Excess weight stresses weight-bearing joints and is thought to be one of the main causes of osteoarthritis in the knees and hips. Every extra pound of weight adds five pounds of excess weight on the hips and knees, increasing wear and tear on the cartilage and causing pain when walking.

Excess weight also causes diminished mobility, which reduces physical activity. We now know that, contrary to prior belief, exercise helps fight joint pain. Any exercise that promotes muscles stretching and blood circulation can ease arthritis pain. Exercise is vital in maintaining joint mobility and can also take the mind off the problem: moving around and doing a physical activity like going for a walk can be distracting enough to help take the focus away from painful joints. And, exercise promotes...weight loss.

Furthermore, we know that cholesterol can clog arteries, seriously compromising blood circulation. Irrigation of muscles and ligaments surrounding joints keeps them in good condition and prevents wear and tear. A diet rich in saturated fats not only causes weight gain, it also increases harmful cholesterol levels.

Finally, some medicines, such as corticosteroids (like prednisone) prescribed to patients with rheumatoid arthritis may cause side effects such as increased appetite, fluid retention and weight gain. The results from this treatment can be disappointing on many levels.

Losing weight is therefore a necessity for any person suffering from arthritis hoping to improve their health. How to do it? Any specialist worth his salt will tell you: exercise and change your diet. It is imperative to diminish sugar and saturated fat intake, but dietary changes must be permanent to avoid the dreaded yo-yo effect associated with fad diets.

The goal of this book is not to offer a weight-loss program for arthritis sufferers; nor does it mean to be restrictive in any way. But it is certainly not a bad thing if almost all of the foods it recommends to fight arthritis are healthy and low in fat and calories. Because of this, it can be a handy reference in establishing a nutritionally-balanced diet that will help you control your weight and stay healthy, whether or not you are obese, as long as portions remain reasonable.

Foods to avoid

Bad fats

The first word of advice in the case of excess weight, is to avoid foods that contain *saturated fats*. This is especially valid for anyone with rheumatoid arthritis, because saturated fats are said to promote inflammation. What are the main sources of saturated fats? Meats are at the top of the list along with other animal-derived foods such as butter and cheese. It is also found in palm oil, palm kernel oil and coconut oil, and in many processed foods. So, be careful and try to cut down on processed foods, particularly deli meats, and above all, read the labels.

A particularly harmful fat is *arachidonic acid*, an unsaturated fat found in meat, egg yolks and dairy products, which is responsible for triggering inflammation-causing free radicals.

Trans fats have been making headlines for a few years now because of their role in increasing bad cholesterol and depleting good cholesterol. And as we know, bad circulation in and around the joints can cause their deterioration. In the food industry, trans fats found in hydrogenated oils give foods such as margarine a solid form. Exercise caution when looking out for the many other foods containing trans fats, especially anything listing shortening as an ingredient (pies, cakes, pastries, muffins, cookies, crackers, chips, etc.). Thankfully, more and more food makers are offering trans fat-free foods, but it is still a good idea to watch out for other fats, salt and sugars used in any given food product.

Questionable foods

Some experts systematically advise arthritis sufferers against many foods, such as red meat and pork, which contain inflammation-causing saturated fatty acids. Processed meats that are smoked and salted, like bacon, ham, sausages and other deli meats, should always be avoided, as they contain preservatives and chemicals that may cause arthritic-like allergic reactions. We can add grapeseed, soy, sunflower, safflower and corn oils, coffee and alcohol to the list. Some of these are only contra-indicated for people suffering from rheumatoid arthritis.

Other foods seem controversial; some reports claim they are responsible for triggering or aggravating arthritis pain, while experts affirm they are either healthy or harmless. In this category, we find dairy products, tomatoes, citrus, peanuts and some grains.

You should not reject generally healthy foods unless recommended by a health professional who is aware of your particular condition. Some confusion appears to be caused by the notion that certain foods may cause joint inflammation as an allergic reaction when it is more of a food intolerance issue.

Food intolerance: where is the culprit?

When looking for a direct link between diet and arthritis, scientists have come to admit that it is possible for some foods to trigger an autoimmune reaction increasing or worsening joint inflammation. This phenomenon appears to affect a small percentage - 5% - of arthritis sufferers.

If you notice that arthritis flare-ups occur regularly after certain meals, it is certainly worth investigating. You may not be allergic to the food in question, but it may be a trigger food in your case. Many nutritionists prefer the term "food intolerance" to "food allergy", insisting that reactions are similar but less severe. What are these trigger foods? They are foods that do not completely break down in the digestive system, leaving undigested particles in the intestinal tract that pass through into the blood stream, provoking an abnormal autoimmune reaction. There are three ways to identify the culprit and all three require discipline. But if a particular food is your trigger, it is certainly worth the effort to eliminate it. Imagine, all you would have to do is never eat that food again to be rid of arthritic pain! Wishful thinking? Maybe, or maybe not...

The first and easiest method is to keep a *food journal.* In one column, write down everything ingested at every meal: liquids and solids. In a second column, write down any reaction in the following hours: increased or diminished pain and any other changes. If you suspect a certain food, do not eat it for two weeks. Never eliminate more than one food at a time. After two weeks, re-introduce the food, making sure to pay attention to any change in symptoms.

The second method is the exclusion *diet formulated by Dr. Irwin,* an American doctor, which also seeks to identify trigger foods in order to avoid them permanently. After rating your pain, you have to follow a basic diet for one week, including foods known to be safe, such as fruit (grape, peach, pear, plum, prune, avocado), vegetables (lettuce, celery, olives, parsley, cauliflower, peas, spinach, squash), rice, olive oil, fish (cod, halibut, salmon, tuna) or turkey, lots of water and salt, if needed. You must eat only these foods for seven days. Be sure to avoid products containing any ingredients other than these foods!

If your pain diminishes or disappears after seven days, or if you have noticed a slight improvement, that means there is a food in your regular diet which does not suit you. The next part of this method consists of re-introducing the foods of your usual diet one at a time. You may chose to re-introduce the foods you suspect to be problematic more rapidly. They may be part of the high-risk group including: citrus, grains (oat, rye, wheat), corn and peanut oil, dairy products, alcohol, coffee and chocolate.

The key to success is to re-introduce each food separately. You must eat that particular food in large quantities for two days in order to provoke an undesirable reaction. This might cause intense pain, but is worth knowing for sure. Then you will know that all you have to do is eliminate the food from your diet to be pain-free. It is important not to make any other changes in your habits or medicines during this test period, or you risk compromising the results.

The third method is a *diet rotation* developed by an American allergist in the 1920s, which has since been revamped and approved by some dieticians. The diet involves formulating three menus for days A, B and C. On day A, you eat only foods that you eat often. On day B, you eat foods that you eat less often. Day C is for foods that you rarely eat. Keeping track of your body's reaction throughout the process (which lasts about three months) will allow you to determine which foods are harmful and which ones you are sensitive to.

It is strongly recommended that you try this method under medical supervision and that you avoid it if you have known allergies.

Learn to know the foods you eat

In order to avoid foods that are harmful, such as foods made with saturated fats and trans fats, or foods that you might be sensitive or allergic to, it is important to understand what you are eating. This is easier to do if you cook your own food, as opposed to eating prepared foods or eating out.

Paradoxically, arthritis sufferers might have a tendency to eat poorly because cooking can be painful and it seems more practical (and faster) to buy prepared foods that you just heat and serve. But this habit can be bad for joint pain (making it worse), as well as for health in general.

It is essential to know what you are buying, to read the labels, and to understand the information on them. However, you should take the time and effort to prepare your own meals by following simple recipes, such as those offered in this book. It is always possible to find ways to minimize movements, but don't forget that exercising your joints is highly recommended.

Foods to choose

We are finally in friendly territory: the foods that are good for arthritis. And good news:

there are many of them! If you have to forgo certain foods and replace them with others, you will be better off in the end. Taking on a new diet, or modifying some of your existing eating habits is an opportunity to discover new foods and new taste sensations that you will want to share with others, because the wide range of arthritis-friendly foods can be beneficial to everyone.

Foods with anti-inflammatory properties

The withdrawal of the famous anti-inflammatory medication, Vioxx, from the market in 2004, put the dangerous side effects of medications in the spotlight. It has long been known that certain anti-inflammatory non-steroidal drugs, such as aspirin, have potentially disastrous effects on the digestive system. What is less known is that nature produces anti-inflammatory foods with no harmful sideeffects. They may not be as powerful as prescription medication but they are highly recommended to arthritis sufferers for their ability to lessen rheumatic inflammation. This ability is characteristic of omega-3 fatty acids that we do not get enough of compared to omega-6 fatty acids. These fats are both essential, but a typical North American diet rich in meat and dairy products is well-stocked in the omega-6 variety, and lacking in the omega-3s. This imbalance compromises good health, particularly as omega-3s reduce the production of prostaglandin, a substance that contributes to the development of arthritis by deteriorating collagen needed in the cartilage that lines our joints.

Omega-3s are part of a large fatty acid family, including alpha-linolenic acid (ALA) which is found primarily in flaxseed as well as in **nut**, **flax**, **canola** and **soy oils**. Other omega-3 fatty acids are found in fatty fish (mackerel, salmon, tuna, herring, sardines, etc. – see page 93 to 101).

It is now possible to buy **omega-3 enriched eggs**. These come from hens fed with grains containing flaxseed and have ten times the omega-3 of ordinary eggs. Just one of these enriched eggs can provide 25 to 35% of your recommended daily intake of omega-3s. But, be careful when eating eggs, as they also contain arachidonic acid, a bad fat that may exacerbate inflammation as mentioned above. Fish oil has the ability to inhibit the adverse effects of arachidonic acid. Omega-3 fatty acids are not the only anti-inflammatory substance found in foods. Here are a few others:

- *Bromelin:* found mainly in **pineapple**. Inhibits the production of inflammation-causing prostaglandin and has a positive effect on the immune system, which explains the pineapple's reputation as a first-rate health food.

- *Curcumin:* an anti-inflammatory found in **turmeric**, and member of the curcuminoids family of powerful antioxidants. Turmeric is an Indian spice used in curries and garam masala (see p. 252). Compounds similar to curcumin are also present in other spices, such as **clove** and **ginger**.

- *S-Adenosyl-L-methionine:* a naturally-occurring molecule easier to remember by its acronym SAMe, it has anti-inflammatory and anti-pain properties. Found mainly in **Brazil nuts** and **sunflower seeds**.

- **Onion**: the onion and its relatives (**garlic, chives, shallot, green onion, leek,** etc.) are also anti-inflammatory, but it is mostly their antioxidant properties that make them highly recommended to fight arthritis (see below).

Analgesic foods

The anti-inflammatory properties of the foods and compounds described above have the power to reduce pain-causing inflammation, but certain plants have a direct analgesic effect similar to aspirin or acetaminophen with less intensity, due to their weaker dosage. Some of these plants are not considered foods but one of them merits mention as it is a food used mainly as a condiment. This food plant is the many varieties of the **red chili pepper**. It contains *capsaicin* which can provoke the body into releasing endorphins. Endorphins are the body's opium, its natural anesthetic. Phytotherapy treatment uses chili peppers in compresses applied to painful joints. There exist therapeutic creams made with capsaicin to soothe arthritic pain. As mentioned above, Brazil nuts and sunflower seeds also have analgesic properties.

Antioxidant foods

For some years now, antioxidants have been getting a lot of attention, especially in relation to cancer. To understand the role of antioxidants, we must first understand what free radicals do. Many body functions are based on a series of chemical reactions in the cells called oxidation. This results in unstable atoms, or whole molecules called free radicals, that try and bond with stable molecules. Free radicals can be a destructive force. This process can be useful as it helps immune system cells react against tumors, bacteria or virus-contaminated cells. But if free radical production becomes excessive over a certain period of time, damage can occur. It can be compared to rust on a car.

Their damage can be considerable: degenerative disease, cancer, hardening of the arteries, cataracts, accelerated aging, Parkinson's disease and...accelerated degenerative joint disease. Free-radicals can also, over time, weaken the immune system, leaving the body vulnerable to infection and attacks from various external sources: pollution, intoxication, radiation, etc. They also play a role in chronic fatigue, muscle pain and loss of intellectual capacity. Free radicals are not only within the body, they are in the environment: in cigarette smoke, in the air, in water, in pollutants – especially those that contaminate our food.

In order to fight free radicals, the body produces its own antioxidants from nutrients like cysteine (an amino-acid), certain minerals (copper, manganese, selenium and zinc) and vitamin B complex. Foods – our area of interest - supply antioxidants directly to the body. The main food sources of antioxidants are *vitamins C* and *E, carotenoids (alpha-carotene, beta-carotene* and *lycopene), flavonoids, glutathiones, zinc* and *selenium.*

Antioxidants act like rust-proofing on metal, or like lemon juice poured on an apple slice to keep it from turning brown; the acidity of the lemon instantly stops the oxidation process, which causes deterioration. Antioxidants are increasingly vital as our environment is getting more polluted by the minute and industrial-grade foods are becoming more and more adulterated. Furthermore, it has been observed that older people are losing their capacity to produce antioxidants.

Antioxidants can stop free radicals from bonding to the bad cholesterol (LDL) which helps prevent atherosclerosis and blood clots. They are excellent for maintaining good heart health. As we age, it becomes increasingly important to include antioxidants in our diet. They help fight rheumatic diseases, slowing down their progression, but they also promote good general health, having a positive effect on longevity, and allowing us to not only live longer, but live healthier.

Here is an overview of all the nutrients mentioned above with their prime foods of source:

- Vitamin C5: best sources in fruit are **guava, papaya, kiwi, citrus, mango, strawberry, star fruit, cantaloupe** and **pineapple**; in vegetables, they are **sweet pepper, broccoli, Brussels sprout, beet** and **kale**.

- Vitamin E: **wheat germ oil, canola oil, sunflower seed, flaxseed, hazelnut, whole grains, tomato paste, nuts, fish eggs, oat bran, wheat bran, avocado, asparagus** and **spinach**.

- Carotenoids: these are plant pigments that give certain fruits and vegetables their color. There are more than 700 of them, but *alpha-carotene, beta-carotene* and *lycopene* have the best antioxidant properties. Beta-carotene, the pigment that gives color to **carrots** and **pumpkins**, is transformed into vitamin A by the body and is important for vision. Lycopene, the red pigment that gives color to **tomatoes** and **red sweet peppers**, has been proven to help prevent prostate cancer.

In studies, other carotenoids such as *beta-cryptoxanthin* and *zeaxanthin* have shown they might diminish the risk of developing rheumatoid arthritis. These pigments are found in most of the same fruits and vegetable as the other carotenoids, particularly in yellow and orange foods. Foods that contain the most beta-cryptoxanthin are: **sweet pepper, pumpkin, squash, persimmon, tangerine** and **papaya**. The most zeaxanthin is found in: **curly kale, spinach**, summer and winter **squash, broccoli, green peas** and **corn**. Among fresh herbs, parsley is rich in vitamin C, and sage contains the most antioxidants.

Vegetables that have a deep green hue are also rich in carotenoids, especially watercress, broccoli and spinach.

- Flavonoids: another family of pigments that give color to fruits and vegetable and have antioxidant properties. They are found mainly in **cabbage, onion, garlic, lettuce** and **sweet pepper**.

- Glutathiones: Important enzymes in the fight against free radicals. Studies have shown that people who have lower levels of these antioxidants are more at risk of developing arthritis. Foods containing this enzyme are **asparagus, cabbage, cauliflower, potato, tomato, avocado, grapefruit, orange, peach** and **watermelon**.

- Zinc: The best food source for this trace element is **wheat germ**. It can also be found in **legumes** and **pumpkin seeds**, as well as in meat and seafood, but these sources are not recommended for arthritis sufferers, with the exception of oysters, which contain the most zinc.

- ◉ Selenium: Another trace element antioxidant found mainly in **Brazil nuts**. I have already mentioned their anti-inflammatory and anti-pain properties; one single nut is all it takes for the recommended daily intake.

Calcium-rich foods

Osteoporosis, the mineral-depleting disease that weakens and deteriorates bone, is thought to be linked to arthritis. Rheumatoid arthritis is thought to contribute to bone loss, as are some medicines prescribed for arthritis, such as cortisone and other corticosteroids. These drugs can impede normal calcium absorption and cause loss of bone density. For this reason, it is essential to absorb enough calcium as a preventative measure.

Milk and dairy products are the most likely sources of calcium, but as these foods are somewhat controversial and not always recommended for arthritis, it is worth looking at other sources. Certain vegetables contain even more calcium than milk; they are: **sesame seeds, cabbage, soy, almonds, parsley, hazelnuts, chickpeas** and **beans**. Sardines (with the bones) are a good animal-based source. Certain kinds of mineral waters contain calcium. Furthermore, many prepared foods are enriched with added calcium, such as rice, tofu, orange juice and breakfast cereals.

It is important to take certain vitamins and *potassium* along with calcium. *Vitamins D and K* facilitate calcium absorption and retention; potassium limits loss of bone calcium by neutralizing acidity. Sunlight is the main source of vitamin D but there are a few food sources: cod liver oil contains a good amount but is not commonly used in cooking and does not taste very good. Fortunately, better tasting fatty fish such as **salmon, mackerel** and **sardines** can do the job. Vitamin K is found in green vegetables like **cabbage, spinach** and **watercress**. Potassium is present in most fruits and vegetables, especially **banana, dried apricot, potato, legumes** and **whole grains**.

Foods rich in essential minerals

Scientists know that people suffering from osteoarthritis are often deficient in minerals other than calcium, especially boron and zinc. Zinc as already been described as an antioxidant. Boron is another important trace element, but the body does not require it in large quantities. It is present in **root vegetables, avocado**, fruit other than **citrus, peanuts** and **wine**.

Healthy foods: raw or cooked?

The many benefits of certain foods illustrates the importance of nutrient combinations. It is possible however, to combine nutrients by eating different foods together. That is why a balanced diet, one that gives the body the ability to fight disease on its own, is made up of a variety of foods of all colors, textures, tastes…and methods of preparation.

This is an area where opinions and ideas abound and sometimes collide – but a few health trends have stood out in recent years. For example, we know that fresh, organic foods, free of contaminants, are healthier and lower the risk of disease. We also know that certain forms of cooking, such as frying or barbecuing can be harmful in the long run, or at least cancel out the nutritional benefits of the foods cooked in these manners.

So, raw or cooked? That is a whole other debate, but one thing is certain: cooking food at high temperatures over a long period of time destroys many of the nutrients they contain. This is not true for all foods – as in the case of the tomato. When cooked, it offers up more antioxidant lycopene. But for most fruits and vegetables, they offer more health benefits if eaten raw. This would explain why the food industry adds all sorts of nutrients to canned and prepared foods that had to be cooked in their processing.

That said, it is evident that cooking quickly, at lower temperatures and with good fats, helps foods retain their natural nutrients, allowing us to eat foods we would not otherwise enjoy (artichoke, potato, green bean, eggplant or legumes for example), and to bring out their full flavors. Many transformed foods are useful in the kitchen and can be healthy such as whole flour and whole wheat pasta.

I believe it is best, not only for health reasons, but also for taste and pleasure, to alternate and use both raw and cooked foods.

Arthritis-friendly diets

There are many diets out there that claim to be good for arthritis. There is even a non-diet which consists simply of fasting. Some experts believe it is possible for short fasts to provide relief. A short break in eating reduces immune system activity thus reducing disease evolution. A 1991 study showed that a fast, followed by a strict vegan diet (no animal-based products), may have a beneficial effect on people suffering from rheumatoid arthritis.

Raw foodists (vegans that only eat raw foods), and living foodists, who eat raw foods, along with grain sprouts and wheat juice, both claim that their diet cures just about everything, including chronic diseases like arthritis. Obviously, this approach is radical and marginal, devoid of any scientific knowledge.

Books are available that offer complete diets for arthritis including weekly menus that must, of course, be repeated over and over again to be successful. But it seems to me that no one is longing for the days when we used to eat the same meal on a given day of the week repeatedly.

Of course, if you know of a food that worsens your condition, you should avoid it, or at least indulge sparingly, if you feel the need to treat yourself. But in general, a varied diet made up of foods known to be arthritis-fighting, along with those you enjoy, will be better for you. Keep trying new foods and new recipes: you will always enjoy the pleasures of eating and you will be happier and healthier while learning to live with your disease.

The Swiss model

I would like to offer, as a guide, a nutrition model that is not a restrictive diet, but a set of recommendations that could be helpful in creating meal menus. It is inspired by the Swiss Society for Nutrition.

● *Oil and fat*

One tablespoon maximum per day of vegetable oil, preferably olive oil to use uncooked in a salad;

One tablespoon maximum per day of vegetable oil, such as canola or olive oil for cooking;

One tablespoon maximum per day of non-hydrogenated margarine for spreading; no more than one fat food per day (i.e. meat, cheese, pastry, chocolate).

● *Sweets – desserts and snacks*

To be eaten only in moderation. Choose sweets made without trans fats.

● *Meat*

No more than twice a week.

● *Fish*

At least twice a week, preferably fatty fish.

● *Eggs*

No more than one or two per week, including eggs incorporated into recipes.

● *Fruit*

At least three servings per day, preferably fresh, to be eaten before meals or in between meals.

● *Vegetables*

At least five servings per day, two or three of them eaten raw.

● *Legumes*

At least two or three servings per week.

● *Milk and dairy products*

To be eaten in moderation, preferably low in fat.

● *Grains and starch*

At least three servings of starch per day (bread, potatoes, rice, pasta, etc.), preferably made from whole grain.

● *Beverages*

Drink lots of water or fresh juices, at least 6 cups per day. No drinks with added sugar.

Alcohol: No more than two glasses of wine or beer per day.

Change your diet, change your life

These recommendations might seem extreme if you have always eaten without any concern for the effects of food on your body. Such a diet is challenging and it is more realistic to use it as inspiration and guidance, not as an actual diet to follow to the letter.

But it is easier than you might think to modify many of your eating habits by taking on new ones that are more in line with these recommendations. All you need is a set desire to improve your health, to be more self-aware, to tap into your imagination and to be minimally disciplined. These changes can come about slowly and gradually, at your own pace.

There is a real advantage to doing it this way: when you see the positive effect of changes in your habits, you will be encouraged to go forward. If you eat less fat, grease, sugar, milk products, prepared foods and meat, you will feel more alert, you will sleep better, you will wake up feeling better, your pain will lessen, you will be ready to undertake the day and feel like moving around more. In short, you will be ready to reclaim control of your life by giving yourself the right to be healthy and providing your body with the nutrition it needs.

The idea of depriving yourself of foods you love might seem difficult at first. But not if you learn to trade in some old favorites for some new and improved ones. You might try substituting greasy fries with oven-roasted potatoes or carrot sticks; eating fresh fruit instead of cake; replacing a meat course with fish or with a nut-based croquette; trying pâté made with mushrooms instead of fatty pork. Many foods can be replaced with nutritional and healthy substitutes that can be surprisingly tasty and satisfying.

The secret to making successful changes lies in the quality of the substitute solutions that will replace old habits. The trick is to make the new foods more appealing than the old ones. When you know that a particular food is bad for you, I am willing to bet that you will be able to find a new one that satisfies your taste buds and your peace of mind, thanks to its health benefits.

Do not compromise the pleasure of eating

Let's be clear, eating less fat is not a punishment. Rich and fatty foods often have an immediate effect on digestion, causing bloating or discomfort. It is relatively easy to reduce the quantity of butter consumed, and even possible to avoid it completely. It is also easy to substitute healthy oils for shortening and fat by using olive oil, which is known to be beneficial as well as delicious. As for fried foods, deli meats and buttery sauces, although delicious, they can leave a bad taste in your mouth, clog the liver and cause indigestion.

Milk is a staple in our diet from childhood on. The same for cheese and eggs These are foods that have always been recommended by health professionals, including nutritionists. However, scientists increasingly suspect that these foods contribute to cardiovascular disease, some cancers and diabetes. Fortunately, many milk-substitutes exist made from rice and soy that can satisfy the taste for milk and cream. Unfortunately, cheese remains unchallenged by any substitution. If, like me, you refuse to eliminate it from your diet, enjoy it in moderation.

The goal here is not to give up all indulgences. If you have a sweet tooth, do not plan on cutting out all sweets cold turkey. I started by cutting out those sweets that seemed the most harmful and were very high in sugar. I gradually replaced them with fruit, whose sugar is much less damaging.

Unless you are vegetarian, the hardest thing to cut back on is meat. I must admit that even though I have been eating a more balanced and healthy diet for five years now, I find it difficult to go without meat for more than three days in a row. But I am proud to say that I have introduced fish and legumes in my diet as alternatives to meat. Truly, it wasn't much of a sacrifice as I love fish and have developed quite a liking for legumes, especially spicy chilis and chickpea and lentil curries. In a nutshell, I have managed to devise meals that give me adequate protein while reducing joint pain, protecting me from other diseases and providing eating pleasure.

Part 2 of this book will be a trove of information on foods that have pain-fighting properties. I urge you to learn about these amazing foods and discover their many virtues. You will want to add them to your diet, not only to treat arthritis, but also to prevent many other diseases.

You will probably notice that vegetables are at the top of the list of good foods (28), followed closely by fruit (18), and then fatty fish (7). I am sure many of these foods are already part of your daily diet. If that is the case, continue enjoying them while introducing those that you might not be as familiar with. Part 3 will provide many ways to prepare these foods with simple and tasty recipes that allow you to make them part of your meals. As we will see throughout this book, variety is key in making these foods part of an effective treatment. If the prospect still seems intimidating, here are a few ideas to renew your daily diet without giving up on all the things you like.

How to cut down on bad fat

As we know, some fats are harmful and aggravate joint pain. It is relatively easy to eat less of them by making better food choices. Choose leaner meats like chicken (without the skin), rabbit, or lean cuts of beef that you will eat without sauces and cooking juices. Replace deli meats with vegetable terrines, and nut or legume spreads.

Avoid ready-to-eat foods and processed foods and try your hand at simple recipes that will also save you money. Gradually cut down on dairy products and cheese, and only eat two eggs a week. Eliminate butter from your diet, replacing it with non-hydrogenated margarine and olive oil for cooking. Choose canola, nut and soy oils over sunflower, corn and peanut oils. Limit pastries, and all foods rich in sugar, as they turn to fat in your body. Replace them with fruit.

Eating less meat

All foods recommended as part of an arthritis-friendly diet are very helpful if you have decided to cut down on meat. Particularly so are fish and legumes, because they provide much-needed protein. Part of the legume family, soy, comes in many different forms: miso, tempeh, tofu and non-hydrated textured protein. The last two are neutral in taste, and will pick up on the flavors of accompanying foods. They can be added to meat dishes to mimic their taste. If you don't like the texture of tofu, try breaking it up with a fork or try using textured soy protein in its place. Rich in protein, nuts are also a good meat substitute. They can be added to most dishes, dips, terrines, pastas, salads, stews and desserts. If you eat out a lot, choose a meatless dish every other time to vary your menu. And if you eat fast food at lunch time, go for the vegetarian pizza instead of the usual all-dressed to reduce calorie-intake. Most fast-food chains now offer good vegetables choices, give them a try once in a while.

Eating more legumes

A good source of fiber and protein, legumes, such as black, red and white kidney beans, lentils and chickpeas, are precious allies to people watching what they eat with little time to spare. Canned, they have all of their nutritional value and are handy to create delicious dishes. They are great in soups, dips, salads, chilis, stews and curries, and require no meat for full flavor and nutrients. Another benefit is that they will leave you feeling full and satisfied without having to eat too much.

If you are not used to them, start by adding them to soups and stews along with meat, then gradually make dishes where they are the star ingredient. Use them with herbs and spices to give them exotic flavors, or add lemon and orange zest to your recipes. You will be surprised to taste new and different flavors that make the ordinary seem extraordinary.

Eating less

In wealthy countries, it is plain to see that obesity has taken on epidemic proportions. Too many people over-eat and then complain about their health and well-being. We live in a market society that pushes over-consumption. Restaurant portions are almost always too large. But how big is the ideal portion? All nutritionists agree, an adult only needs a small portion of meat, fish or poultry per day--a portion being equal in size to a pack of playing cards. That is usually less than what most people eat. Advertising entices us to snack continually and to eat way more than is needed. It is definitely possible to eat less without feeling deprived or hungry, we just need to eat better.

We should avoid salty foods which can be quite addictive. If you usually snack in between meals, substitute chips and salted peanuts with crudités or fresh fruit. They should calm your appetite enough to get you to the next meal. A plate of raw veggies before a meal will cut down your appetite

and load you up with vitamins, while neutralizing the effect of fat. Hearty soups are good low-calorie starters that are better for you than deli meats and puff pastry.

Eating slowly and chewing enough are other ways to cut down on food intake. These are all little things we should do in order to develop a more healthy and balanced relationship with our food.

Give yourself permission to cheat once in a while but don't go overboard. If this new and improved diet works for you, you should not feel the need to stray off the path very often. On the contrary, if you are feeling the positive effects healthy foods are giving your body, avoiding the foods that cause pain should be easy - especially since you will have discovered the pleasure of eating good foods that you have prepared yourself.

Before moving on to the kitchen, let's take a closer look at all the benefits these foods provide, other than relieving arthritis pain. Part 2 will group them in categories and present them individually with their benefits, and the different ways they can be used in food preparation.

Part Two

Arthritis-fighting foods

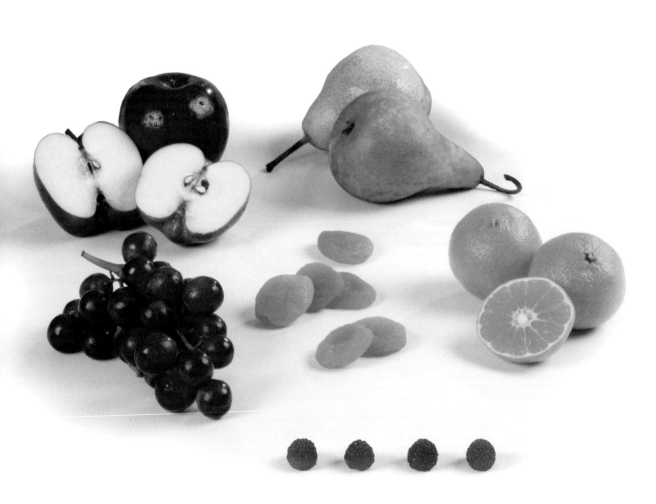

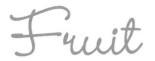
Fruit

Because of the sugar they contain, fruits are more popular than vegetables, making them easier to fit into a balanced diet aimed at improving health. Their high beta-carotene content makes them particularly beneficial to arthritis sufferers along with their vitamin C and fiber content.

Fruit before or after a meal?

Fruits are acidic and the carbohydrates they contain both stimulate and help maintain healthy, regular digestion. That is why they ferment when consumed at the end of a meal. Consequently, it is recommended that people who have problems with bloating and gas eat them before. or in between meals.

Fruit does not produce molecules that are toxic or dangerous to your health, so anyone who tolerates them well at the end of a meal can continue doing so.

Cooking with fruit

A great many traditional cuisines add fruits to their recipes. They go very well with vegetables in a salad and are delicious with meat in stews and other sauce-based dishes. However, like vegetables, they are best consumed fresh and plain to get the most out of them.

Which fruit to pick?

Color is your best guide. The more colorful the fruit, the better it is: blueberries, plums, oranges, red grapes, pink grapefruit, etc. Why is that? Because the antioxidant vitamins A & C they contain in large quantities help reduce joint inflammation. The most recent North American dietary recommendations on daily intake of antioxidants state that it is better to eat a diet rich in fruits and vegetables than to take vitamin and mineral supplements.

How to eat more fruit

Start at breakfast by replacing your reconstituted juice by freshly-squeezed. It takes no more time to squeeze an orange, grapefruit, mandarin or clementine as it does to mix up a can of frozen concentrate, and you can try a different flavor every day of the week. Once you've tasted fresh-squeezed juice, you won't want to go back to ready-made versions and you will get loads of vitamins to boot. Save time by using a blender and add soy milk to your fruit. Again, the combinations you can mix up are limitless. Prepare quick compotes by mixing fresh fruit and honey to accompany your morning toast.

No time for breakfast? Did you know that one kiwi contains more vitamin C than an orange? If you're pressed for time, grab a fruit for a healthy snack alternative. Enhance your vegetable salads by adding some fruit - diced pineapple and pieces of melon and mango. Add dried fruit to your meat or vegetable stews. If you're really in a rush, most grocery stores sell fresh fruit that is already peeled, sliced and packaged for your convenience. After a particularly rich meal, choose fruit instead of cake for dessert.

I highly recommend adding fruit to any crudité platter served as an appetizer as they are easier to digest when eaten before a meal.

The top arthritis-fighting fruits

Apricot

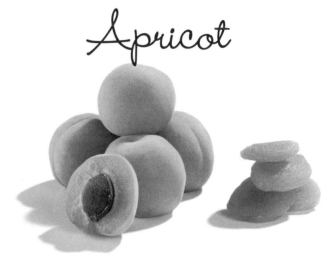

This delicious and nutritious fruit is best when eaten very ripe. Carotene gives it a lovely orange hue and makes it perfect for arthritis sufferers. Beta-carotene ,which is found in many plant food sources, has antioxidant and immunostimulant properties. Apricots also contain lots of potassium, a known anemia-fighting agent. Apricots are as effective as veal liver in the treatment of anemia.

Other health benefits
- Helps prevent cancers of the lungs, pancreas and skin
- Refreshing
- Prevents diarrhea
- Alleviates depression and insomnia

Uses
Eat four slivers of dried apricot every day before breakfast to ease joint pain.

Precautionary warning

Apricots may cause asthma attacks! People allergic to aspirin should avoid apricots. The seed inside the apricot's pit can cause discomfort and can be poisonous if eaten in large quantities.

Buying and storing

Choose a nice golden-orange colored fruit. Touches of red generally indicate it will be sweeter. Like other fruit, keep at room temperature until fully ripened, then store in your fridge.

In the kitchen

Before cooking dried apricot, soak in water, green tea, or fruit juice (apple or orange) until tender. Add to your meat stews along with other dried fruit, such as raisins and figs, or with nuts. Can also be served as a condiment after simmering 20 minutes with other dried fruit like figs, raisins or prunes. Delicious as a compote or dried fruit salad; great to garnish a cake. Apricots are also a tasty snack choice.

Recipes

- Kiwi compote with tea and ginger (p. 130)
- Quick tea jam (p. 132)
- Duck legs with dried fruit (p. 224)

Good to know

Fresh apricot has fewer calories than dried apricot. However, dried apricot contains more beta-carotene than fresh apricot.

Pineapple

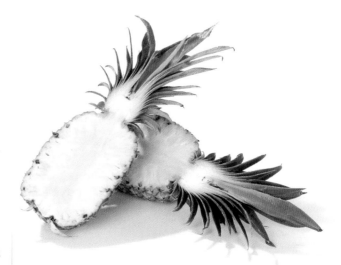

Pineapple contains vitamin C, beta-carotene, potassium and manganese, a little-known mineral useful in fighting free radicals. But its high bromelin content is the reason it excels in treating arthritis pain. Bromelin is an enzyme that breaks down protein and helps digestion.

Other health benefits

- Antiseptic
- Antioxidant, offering protection against cancer and aterosclerosis
- Fights cellulite
- Diuretic
- Facilitates digestion and cleans the digestive tract
- Good for sore throats and cold symptoms
- Relieves heartburn

Uses

Add pineapple cubes to your warm or cold salads.

Precautionary warning

Pineapple can release histamines, like strawberries and tomatoes, possibly causing redness similar to hives for some people. This is not an allergic reaction, but merely indicates a food intolerance. Simply stop eating for symptoms to disappear.

Buying and storing

Pineapple is one the rare fruits that stops ripening when picked. A ripe fruit is heavy, with a discernable scent and green leaves. Do not buy discolored fruit with soft skin. The leaves of a fully-ripened pineapple will tear off easily. Once the skin is cut off, the pineapple will keep in the fridge for a few days. Many fruit markets and grocers sell peeled and cored pineapple.

In the kitchen

Served in slices to be eaten plain, or combined with yogurt, pineapple is a simple and refreshing dessert. It goes well with avocado or spinach in a salad.

Recipe

☐ Fruit salad with curry (p. 265)

Good to know

Because of the protein-breaking bromelin it contains, pineapple is an excellent marinade that tenderizes meat and poultry for grilling. 100 grams of pineapple contains 100 mg of bromelin.

Avocado

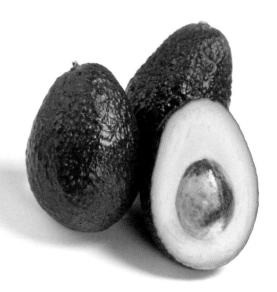

The avocado tree can grow to 50 feet and gives the fruit its amazing properties. Don't be fooled by its rough exterior – it used to be referred to as alligator pear – its deliciously creamy flesh brings youth and beauty to skin thanks to its high vitamin E content. Its monounsaturated fats help reduce cholesterol level, but its glutathione content, an antioxidant known to relieve joint pain, is what makes it a food of choice for treating arthritis.

Other health benefits

- Lowers hypertension
- Helps fight against HIV
- Prevents cellular aging
- Relieves constipation

Precautionary warning

The oil contained in avocado appears to be incompatible with warfarin, a prescription drug that prevents blood clots. People watching their weight should eat it in moderation because even though the fat contained in avocados is beneficial, at 30 grams it is worth half of the recommended daily intake for the average person.

Buying and storing

Avocado continues to ripen after being picked and only keeps for few days at room temperature. Once the skin blackens and the flesh feels soft, it is ripe and ready to eat. It can be kept a bit longer if stored in the fridge once ripe.

In the kitchen

Its delicate flavor make it a delectable entrée in a cold soup, in a dip, or to accompany salmon, crab or shrimp. It is best served raw, as cooking will make it bitter. It can also be cubed and added to a salad or combined with fruit.

Recipes

- Stuffed avocado infused with lemon and curry (p. 160)
- Grapefruit, avocado and fennel cup (p. 170)
- Melon and avocado salad (p. 168)

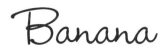

Banana

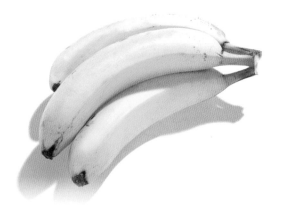

The Latin name for bananas means "fruit of the wise", which might explain why it is reputed to be good for all, from babies to the elderly. It is an excellent source of vitamin C and potassium, a mineral beneficial to arthritis sufferers. Athletes also appreciate its nourishing calories, as it delivers the kind of carbohydrates that are the most efficient at developing muscles mass.

Other health benefits

- Cures diarrhea
- Promotes bone growth and health
- Protects the nervous system
- Lowers hypertension

Uses

Eating one banana a day is recommended for people who have a sensitive stomach and frequent indigestion.

Precautionary warning

Bananas should be eaten fully ripe for their digestive and healing properties to be at their best. Its Caribbean cousin, the plantain, should be cooked. Because it is rich in carbohydrates, the banana is not recommend for diabetics, or for people trying to lose weight.

Buying and storing

Choose nice bright yellow fruit without bruising that will ripen quickly.

In the kitchen

Eaten raw and plain, or sliced in a bowl of cereal, the banana is a tasty and nutritious breakfast. It's also great for snacks and is wonderful in fruit salads or blended in fruit juices.

Recipe

❑ Banana and clementine smoothie (p. 134)

Good to know

The black ink-like blotches on its skin will disappear when rubbed with the inside of a banana peel.

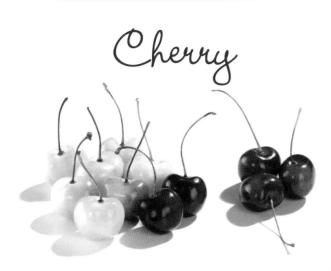

Cherry

Even though it is rich in sugar, the cherry is still recommended for diabetics and obese people because the kind of sugar it contains, fructose, is assimilated into the bloodstream. This delicious fruit is a perfect appetite-suppressant, full of vitamins and minerals. It is commonly believed to cure gout and rheumatism and studies have seen evidence that it does, indeed, relieve these conditions.

Other health benefits

- Ensures good intestinal function
- Purifying and detoxifying properties
- Diuretic
- Lowers risk of cardiovascular disease
- Hepatic and gastric regulator
- Relieves gout

Home remedy

Anti-gout recipe

Put a handful of cherry stems in a pot with 4 cups of boiling water. Lower heat and let simmer for 7 to 10 minutes. Remove from heat and let sit, covered, for 20 minutes. Drink 2 cups a day.

Precautionary warning

Avoid drinking water after eating cherries because this will cause the cellulose in your stomach to bloat.

Raw cherries are not recommended for people with dyspepsia (chronic indigestion) and for people with sensitive stomachs; they should eat them in compotes or jams. Cherries should not be eaten in large amounts by people wanting to lose weight, as they are high in calories and, being addictive, it is difficult to eat just a few.

Buying and storing

Bigaroon cherries are firm and sweet, with a deep red color. Sour cherries are tart, as their name implies, and are yellowish pink or light red. The stems should be green; dark stems indicate lack of freshness. Do not wash cherries before storing them in your fridge but make sure you do before eating.

In the kitchen

Cherries are good in jams but cooking robs them of their nutritional value so eating them raw is preferable. Juice is another good use. Some health food stores sell organic cherry juice that is supposed to preserve all of this fruit's virtues.

Recipe

❑ Quinoa with cherries and nuts (p. 238)

Good to know

In order to enjoy them all year round, you may freeze cherries, making sure to pit them first. Spread them out on a cookie sheet much like you would for berries, in a single layer, and put the sheet in the freezer for a few hours. Then store them in airtight containers where they will keep in the freezer for up to 6 months. You can also dry them and keep them up to one year stored in the pantry in an airtight container.

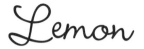

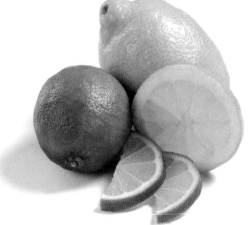

With its zesty flavor and bright color, the lemon owes its medicinal reputation to its high concentration of vitamin C. It also contains carotene, mineral salts and oligo elements. Its antioxidant properties prevent joint pain progression. It is also helpful in eliminating uric acid, which worsens joint pain. Not only are the juice and rind of the lemon very useful in cooking, this fruit also lends a helping hand cleaning up the kitchen.

Other health benefits

- Relieves and treats gastric problems
- Contains remineralizing substances
- Prevents colds and relieves cold symptoms
- Refreshingly tonic
- Treats anemia
- Anti-parasitic

Home remedy

Steep a slice of lemon in one cup of hot water to drink after a meal; it will purify the blood by eliminating toxins.

Precautionary warning

Best when ripe. The rind or zest gives a nice flavor to salads, vinaigrettes, meat stews, fish, pasta and cakes – but make sure it is pesticide-free. It is usually sprayed with wax to preserve its color. If you cannot find organic lemons, scrub lemons thoroughly, or let them soak in warm water for a few seconds (or a few hours in cold water) to dissolve the wax coating. As soon as the juice comes in contact with air, the vitamins will oxidize and lose their properties. The same is true for oranges and grapefruit. To take full advantage of citrus benefits, drink the juice as soon as it is squeezed from the fruit.

Buying and storing

Choose firm, ripe fruits with a fine-grained rind, untreated if available. Store in a cold dark place.

In the kitchen

Whether raw or cooked, the lemon is very useful in cooking because all parts are edible. It gives unbelievable flavor to all dishes, sweet or savory. Its uses are many: in vinaigrettes, replace the vinegar with lemon juice and add a touch of grated lemon zest. To get the most out of this antioxidant fruit, put a few sections, including the white membrane, in the blender when preparing juices and smoothies.

Recipes

Good to know

A round lemon is usually juicier than an oval lemon.

Hard-shelled fruit (nuts)

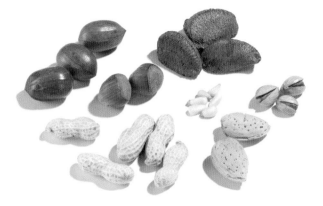

*n*uts are hard-shelled fruit that all belong to the same family. The most commonly used are: almond, peanut, cashew, chestnut, macadamia, hazelnut, Brazil nut, pecan, pistachio.

These fruits used to have a bad reputation, due to their high fat and calorie content. Research now indicates that they may diminish the risk of cardiovascular disease because the fats they contain are the "good" kinds – poly-unsaturated and mono-unsaturated - that lower cholesterol. They also contain protein, fiber, copper, magnesium, phytosterols and antioxidants – all substances that play a role in relieving and preventing joint pain. Furthermore, Brazil nuts contain selenium, an important antioxidant with known anti-inflammatory properties.

Other health benefits

- Antidiarrheal and laxative
- Ensure good intestinal function
- Prevent cardiovascular disease
- Protect against cancer

Home remedy

Eating one Brazil nut a day provides the daily recommended intake of selenium. When you foresee a day of strenuous physical activity, try this tonic recipe: in a blender, pour one glass of a juice of your choice, add a handful of nuts, and mix. But be careful not to overindulge or drink it every day if you are counting calories.

Uses

Eating nuts in small quantities to replace less healthy fatty snacks like cookies and chips, is an excellent way to enjoy their health benefits.

Health tip

To make nuts easier to digest, soak them in water overnight in the fridge. They will then be quite a bit softer.

Precautionary warning

Nuts can cause allergies. Because they are so rich in fats, nuts must be eaten in small quantities, especially if they are gradually substituted in place of other caloric foods.

Peanuts can cause severe allergic reactions resulting in anaphylactic shock and even death.

Buying and storing

Nuts are available shelled, chopped or ground. It is best to buy them in a store that does brisk business because they go rancid quite quickly. Choose proportionately heavy nuts and store them in airtight containers in a cool dark place. They freeze well when whole and don't require defrosting before use.

In the kitchen

Nuts have a sweet, tangy flavor that goes well with vegetables in a stir-fry or salad; together they make a satisfying meal. They are also delicious in desserts and are a flavorful addition to tofu and grains.

Recipes

- Asparagus with orange and pecans (p. 158)
- Hazelnut and pecan burgers (p. 182)
- Squash stuffed with salmon, rice and pine nuts (p. 176)
- Lemon couscous with pistachios and pine nuts (p. 234)
- Apple crisp with ginger and pecans (p. 266)
- Trout with almond tartar sauce (p. 209)
- Fusilli with cauliflower and cherry tomatoes (pine nuts) (p. 190)
- Macaroni au gratin with mushrooms and cashews (p. 190)
- Green beans with lemon and almonds (p. 236)
- Rabbit with dried fruit (hazelnut) (p. 226)

- Liver pâté (pistachios) (p. 228)
- Mini lasagna rolls with pistachios and artichoke hearts (p. 197)
- Quick fruit and lentil picadillo with golden pita (almonds) (p. 193)
- Basil and pistachio pesto (p. 251)
- Quick winter pesto (pecans) (p. 251)
- Pizza with goat cheese and pesto (pecans) (p. 178)
- Cherry and nut quinoa (cashews) (p. 238)
- Apple- and orange-flavored rice (pistachios) (p. 241)
- Endive and fennel salad with apple (hazelnuts) (p. 169)
- Papaya, mango and kiwi salad infused with vanilla (pine nuts) (p. 166)
- Spaghetti with zucchini and hazelnuts (p. 194)
- Salmon imperial triangles (almonds) with mushroom and pistachio variations (p. 161)

Good to know

Walnuts and almonds contain the most vitamin E of any food except for edible oils. Almonds, walnuts and hazelnuts contain 44 to 61 mg of calcium per 100 grams, making them richer in calcium than milk.

Persimmon

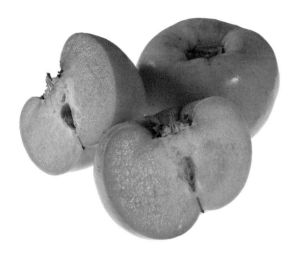

A lso called kaki fruit, the persimmon is better known in Europe than in America. It is among the high energy fruits like cherries and grapes. Its high vitamin C content make it ideal for arthritis sufferers. It has a high beta-carotene content along with other pigments, like the lycopene that gives it its vibrant orange color, which protect the immune system by attacking free radicals. The potassium it contains helps limit calcium loss thereby protecting bone structure.

Other health benefits
◦ Helps prevent infection

Home remedy
To help ward off the flu, use a blender to mix up a healthy concoction made with one persimmon and one kiwi, peeled.

Buying and storing
The tannins which give the persimmon a slight astringency diminish as the fruit ripens, at the same time its sugar level rises. It should be eaten at its peak, when it has lost some of its acridity and its beauty. It is then not quite as appealing-looking, with a discolored almost translucent skin, but it will be delicious and quite fragile. Once ripe, it will keep in the produce compartment of your fridge for a few days - no longer than two days if overripe. To hasten the ripening process, put it with some apples in a fruit basket at room temperature.

In the kitchen
Slice it or cube it to add an exotic touch to fruit salads and green salads. Pureed, it makes wonderful sorbet, mousse and jam. It goes very well with quark cheese and yogurt.

Good to know
Persimmon is extremely popular in Japan. The Japanese love to eat it tempura-style to accompany shrimp.

Kiwi

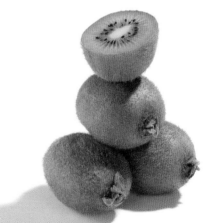

D on't be fooled by its unattractive brown fuzzy appearance, once sliced its beautiful emerald vitamin C-loaded flesh is revealed. Low in fat and sodium, the kiwi contains lots of potassium, which makes it a perfect fruit for arthritis sufferers. The kiwi is the fruit that offers the highest density of nutrients.

Other health benefits

- Lowers cholesterol
- Fights hypertension
- Alleviates cold symptoms
- Prevents cancer

Uses

You can easily replace your morning glass of orange juice with a peeled kiwi for a mega-dose of vitamin C.

Precautionary warning

No contra-indications are known, so enjoy at will!

Buying and storing

Choose unblemished fruit that is not too hard or dried up. A ripe kiwi smells pleasingly of banana and lime and has a little give to the touch.

In the kitchen

The kiwi is eaten fresh and plain; its gorgeous emerald color is quite decorative in a fruit salad. It goes very well with fish and grilled meat.

Recipes

- Kiwi compote with tea and ginger (p. 130)
- Papaya, mango and kiwi salad infused with vanilla (p. 166)

Good to know

Gram for gram, the kiwi contains more vitamin C than any citrus: 100 grams of kiwi provides a full daily adult intake.

Mango

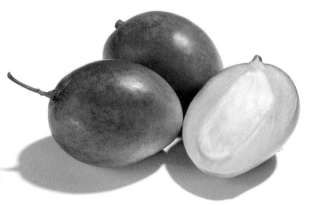

The uber-refreshing mango is the third most popular fruit in the world, after the banana and citrus fruits. There are over 500 varieties of mango. Rich in beta-carotene, vitamins B & C, calcium and potassium, it is also the fruit that contains the most vitamin A, making it one the better fruits for arthritis sufferers.

Other health benefits

- Fights skin disease
- Lowers risk of cardiovascular disease
- Prevents cell aging
- Protects against certain types of cancers

Uses

Eating one to two mangos a week will prevent joint pain with the added bonus of keeping skin soft and supple.

Precautionary warning

Mango skin can be irritating to the mouth so it is best to peel it before eating.

Buying and storing

A ripe mango has a pleasant smell and slight give to the touch. Avoid hard or wrinkly fruit. Keep it out of the fridge: a true tropical fruit, it hates the cold! Unripe mango will take about a week to ripen at room temperature.

In the kitchen

Mango is best enjoyed plain, its flesh scooped out with a spoon. Cubed, it is delicious in fruit or vegetable salads. It goes very well with shrimp, pork and chicken.

Recipes

- Instant mango cream (p. 260)
- Curried fruit salad (p. 265)
- Mango and watercress salad (p. 170)
- Papaya, mango and kiwi salad infused with vanilla (p. 166)

Good to know

The darker the mango's flesh, the higher its vitamin A content.

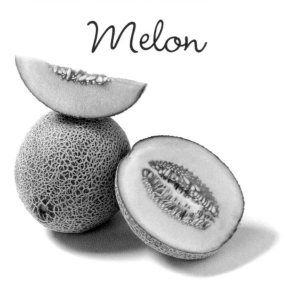

Melon

elon is not only delicious, it is packed with healthy nutrients. There are many varieties of melon, but the most popular are cantaloupe and musk melon. Fortunately, these are in fact the melons that offer the most value for arthritis sufferers because of their high content in vitamin C, beta-carotene, mineral salts and folates.

Other health benefits

- Lowers blood pressure
- Anticoagulant
- Refreshing
- Fights anemia
- Diuretic
- Laxative
- Refreshing
- Rejuvenates tissue
- Lowers cancer risk
- Prevents cataracts

Home remedy

Thanks to melon's high beta-carotene content, arthritis sufferers notice joint-pain improvement when they eat a slice of cantaloupe before every meal.

Precautionary warning

Melon is not recommended for diabetics and for people with enteritis (inflammation of the intestines) and dyspepsia (chronic digestive problems).

Buying and storing

Choose a heavy, unblemished fruit. Melon does not ripen after harvest: look for a fruit that has a slight depression where the stem was attached indicating maturity. A ripe melon has a nice smell; if the smell is too strong, the melon is overripe and about to ferment. Avoid melons that do not smell enough and those that smell too strongly.

In the kitchen

Italians know what they are doing when serving melon as an entrée; that is how to get the most health benefits. Add melon to your lettuce or cabbage salads for a visual - and flavorful – punch.

Recipes

- ☐ Honeydew and strawberry smoothie (p. 134)
- ☐ Cantaloupe and grape salad with ginger (p. 158)
- ☐ Curried fruit salad (p. 265)
- ☐ Melon and avocado salad (p. 168)

Good to know

As with most fruit, it is best to eat melon before a meal. Salt and pepper will make it easier to digest.

Orange

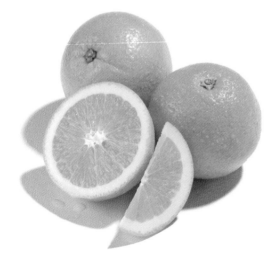

$\mathcal{W}$ith its round shape and sun-like color, is it any wonder that the juicy orange packs so many healthy nutrients? It offers a generous helping of vitamin C, which has many beneficial properties such as fighting bacteria, viruses and many forms of inflammation.

Other health benefits

- ☻ Protects against hemorrhage
- ☻ Protects against infection
- ☻ Refreshing
- ☻ Lowers risk of cardiovascular disease
- ☻ Fights against certain types of cancer
- ☻ Purifies the blood
- ☻ Cell and skin rejuvenating
- ☻ Boosts natural defenses
- ☻ Relieves asthma

Home remedy

A glass of fresh-squeezed orange juice each morning is an excellent way to protect against various infections because the juice has as much vitamin C as the fruit itself, if consumed as soon as it's squeezed.

Uses

Daily consumption of oranges provides energy, purifies the blood and acts as an antiseptic. To benefit from the orange's arterial protection, it must be eaten whole - pulp and membrane included - as they contain the pectin that does the job.

Precautionary warning

Oranges can trigger a condition called "oral allergy syndrome" which causes itching and burning in the mouth and throat. This is a rare allergy and its symptoms will dissipate quickly if you stop eating the trigger food.

Buying and storing

Oranges will keep for more than a week at room temperature and even longer in the fridge.

In the kitchen

The orange is one of those fruits that can be served from the entrée all the way through to dessert. It can be sliced thinly or split into sections and added to salads. It's great in pies, yogurt and cakes. Its juice and grated zest infuse wonderful flavor to sautéed and stewed dishes made up of meat or fish, grilled foods, rice and couscous, vinaigrettes and marinades.

Recipes

- Asparagus with orange and pecans (p. 158)
- Orange-infused beets (p. 234)
- Apple crisp with ginger (p. 266)
- Rabbit à l'orange with ginger (p. 228)
- Clementine and carrot salad with sage (p. 160)
- Clementine and turmeric sauce (p. 130)
- Orange and curry vinaigrette (p. 246)

Good to know

Commercially-prepared orange juice is not as nutritious as freshly-squeezed. Recent studies have shown that supermarket varieties of orange juice have no anti-viral properties.

Grapefruit

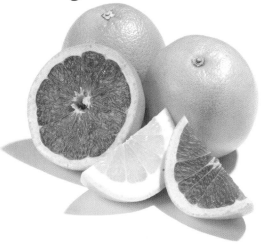

Like other citrus fruit, grapefruit is rich in vitamins A & C and mineral salts. But it also contains rheumatoid-fighting substances all its own. Research has shown that the pectin in grapefruit neutralizes the harmful effects of a fatty diet.

Other health benefits

- Protects against hemorrhage
- Refreshing
- Lowers risk of cancer
- Digestive and diuretic
- Promotes healing of lesions
- Lowers cholesterol (the fruit)
- Relieves cold symptoms

Uses

Before over-indulging or eating rich foods, peel and enjoy a beautiful pink grapefruit; this will help prevent clogging of the arteries.

Precautionary warning

Grapefruit and grapefruit juice (fresh or frozen) contain substances that may have an effect on how certain medications are absorbed and transformed. If you take any medication, consult your doctor or pharmacist to see if any interaction is contra-indicated before consuming grapefruit of any kind. Cutting a grapefruit in half to empty out the pulp will cause it to lose many nutrients, as half of its pectin is in the membrane. The best way to eat it is to peel and enjoy.

Buying and storing

Choose a heavy and firm fruit. Pink grapefruit contains the most lycopene, the powerful antioxidant capable of neutralizing free radicals, so go for the more colorful varieties such as ruby red, ruby and star ruby.

In the kitchen

Grapefruit is excellent in salads and, combined with other fruits, can make delicious desserts.

Recipe

 Grapefruit, avocado and fennel cup (p. 170)

Tasty trick

Yummy citrus drink
Tone down the grapefruit's acidity by combining it with other, sweeter citrus fruit, such as oranges and clementines, or any other sweet fruit. In a blender, mix grapefruit sections with 2 oranges and 2 clementines. Then add 20 or so strawberries and blend again.

Good to know

Relatively low in pectin, grapefruit juice does not lower blood cholesterol. To benefit from all its properties, it should be eaten whole, including the white membrane. Pink grapefruit contains as much vitamin C as white grapefruit but has twice the beta-carotene.

Berries
Blueberry — cranberry — strawberry — raspberry

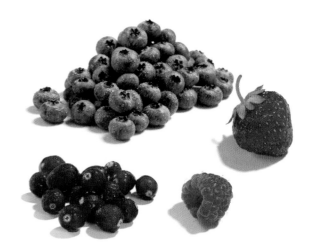

The **blueberry** is a tiny fruit that does not contain many nutrients but is excellent for dessert due to its high fiber content. Like other berries, it does contain vitamin C, an important antioxidant in the prevention of cataracts and eye infections.

The **cranberry** contains an antibiotic that protects the bladder – like blueberry juice – and controls bacteria.

The **strawberry** is rich in vitamins and mineral salts. Because its sugar is fructose, it is recommended for diabetics. It also contains glutathione, an antioxidant that has been proven to slow down deterioration of the immune system. Along with the kiwi, the strawberry shares the title of the fruit richest in vitamin C.

Rich in vitamins B & C, potassium and various acids, the **raspberry** is a delight even diabetics and arthritis sufferers can enjoy because the fructose it contains has no harmful effects. It is low in calories and rich in fiber making it a good constipation remedy.

Other health benefits

- Accelerates intestinal activity (raspberry)
- Antidiabetic (blueberry, cranberry)
- Improves vision (blueberry, cranberry)
- Astringent, antiseptic, anti-putrid (blueberry, strawberry, raspberry)
- Helps prevent cancer and degenerative diseases (blueberry)
- Fights HIV (strawberry)
- Purifying (strawberry, raspberry)
- Lowers risk of cardiovascular disease (raspberry)
- Diuretic (strawberry, raspberry)
- Prevents constipation (strawberry)
- Prevents and treats urinary conditions such as cystitis (cranberry)
- Protects against cell aging (raspberry)
- Protects vascular walls (blueberry)
- Relieves vascular insufficiency (blueberry)
- Relieves diarrhea (blueberry)
- Relieves gout (strawberry)
- Relieves stomach discomfort (raspberry)
- Treats inflammation of mucous membrane of the mouth (blueberry, raspberry)

Uses

- It is recommended to eat **blueberries** every day as an appetizer before a meal.
- Added to breakfast cereal, **raspberries** are an excellent source of fiber and help in protecting against cardiovascular disease.
- Two small glasses of **cranberry** juice per day – about ½ cup – protect against urinary tract infections.

Precautionary warning

Cooking causes **blueberries** to lose their healing properties, so it is best to eat them raw.

Diabetics should take **cranberry** extract in pill-form or drink pure cranberry juice, as many of the cranberry cocktail-type drinks available in stores are loaded with sugar.

Strawberries are not recommended for people suffering from dermatitis; they can cause allergies and benign skin breakouts that will disappear as soon as you stop eating it.

People with sensitive intestines should use **raspberries** as a coulis that can be strained to remove the seeds that might be problematic to them.

Buying and storing

Choose firm **blueberries** that are a pretty matte blue. Do not wash before refrigerating uncovered, and use them promptly as they will only last two days in the fridge. Once washed and dried, they can be frozen to be used in cooking and baking. To freeze, spread them out on a cookie sheet and put them in the freezer until hardened before putting them in an airtight container.

Look for plump, firm **cranberries** that are bright red in color. Wash them only when ready to use; they will keep longer--up to two months--in the fridge.

Do not choose **strawberries** that have white on them; they will not ripen. Strawberries are best eaten soon after picking, but will keep for a few days if sprinkled with sugar and stored in the fridge. They can also be frozen in the same manner as blueberries.

Raspberries keep for a short time in the fridge. They are very delicate so wash only just before eating.

In the kitchen

Blueberries are tasty and versatile, from snacks to breakfast, in puddings, cakes, clafoutis, sorbets, jellies and anything kind of desserts. To enjoy fresh, rinse them in water with a teaspoon of vinegar added.

Because of their tart flavor, it is best to cook **cranberries** rather than eat them raw. They can then be used in cakes, cookies and muffins. Cook them in a bit of water but keep them covered; the heat will cause them to swell and burst. They are delicious in chutney, compote, jam or jelly. Dried cranberries are perfect in your breakfast cereal.

Serve plain fresh **strawberries** for dessert. They are delicious in jam and perfect for pies and cakes. Add them to your tossed salad for a refreshing and daringly new twist. They are also available dried making them easy to add to cereal or any kind of vegetable salad.

Served plain, **raspberries** are a wonderful snack and a real delight with a dollop of yogurt.

Recipes
- Quick tea jam (strawberries and dried cranberries) (p. 132)
- Honeydew and strawberry smoothie (p. 134)

Good to know
Berries retain a large amount of pesticide residue; it is recommended to buy organic. Recent Canadian studies have found that **cranberry** extract fights certain intestinal viruses. Scientists are trying to determine if those same chemical substances could be as efficient in other parts of the body.

A 100-gram portion of **strawberries** contains almost the entire daily recommended intake of vitamin C.

The leaves of the **raspberry** plant have astringent, diuretic and laxative properties. In some Anglo-Saxon countries, raspberry leaf tea is administered to women in labour.

Papaya

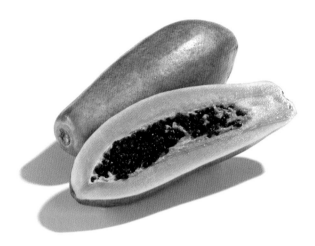

The sweet juicy papaya is similar to melon and particularly rich in vitamins A, B & C, mineral salts and trace elements including potassium, calcium and magnesium which helps neuromuscular function and protects bone. It is rich in beta-carotene with 100 grams of flesh providing 30% of the daily required intake. The deeper the color, the higher the nutrient content.

Other health benefits
- Digestive
- Lowers risk of cardiovascular disease
- Skin firming

Uses
It is a perfect food for the sick and aged who will benefit from its nutritious and digestive qualities and easy-to-swallow flesh. It can be used raw or cooked with other refreshing fruits for a nice entrée or a delicious dessert.

Precautionary warning

Ripe papaya is soft, with easy to tolerate, melt-in-the-mouth goodness. However, some people with sensitive stomachs should eat it as a blended coulis.

Buying and storing

Papaya is ripe when it offers a little give to the touch. If it needs to ripen, let it stand at room temperature. If you want to hasten the ripening process, wrap it in a paper bag as you would an avocado. Some fruit stores will sell halved papayas.

In the kitchen

Eat papaya raw like a melon. When it is still green, it can be boiled or cooked in fruit juice to be served as compote.

Recipe

☐ Papaya, mango and kiwi salad infused with vanilla (p. 166)

Good to know

Papain, the milk substance contained in the fruit has long been familiar to Africans who use it to tenderize meat before cooking.

Pear

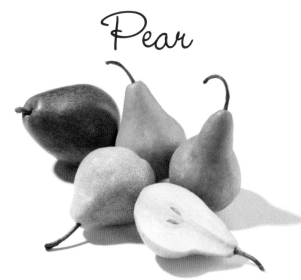

The pear tree offers a delicious fruit filled with nutrients, mineral salts and B vitamins. Diabetics can include it in their diet because it contains levulose, a fruit sugar they can eat. Pear is particularly recommended for arthritis sufferers; it contains a precious mineral – boron – that stops calcium loss, helping to keep bones healthy. Boron has the added property of stimulating intellectual faculties and protecting against age-related memory loss.

Other health benefits

- Lowers cholesterol
- Diuretic
- Protects against colon cancer
- Stimulates the brain

Uses

Pear is available most of the time, so it would be a shame not to take advantage of this delicious fruit that has so much to offer. Two pears are all it takes to get 32% of the recommended daily intake of fiber. Furthermore, pear is said to clear the complexion and give smooth, radiant skin to those who eat it.

Precautionary warning

It is best to eat pear unpeeled because most of its fiber is in the outer skin. However, make sure to wash it thoroughly first.

Buying and storing

There are hundreds of varieties of pear all over the world. Our markets carry mostly the Anjou, Bartlett, Bosc and Comice varieties. Like the avocado, pear does not mature well on the tree and will continue to ripen and develop its flavor after being picked. However, it will ripen in a few days, and then turn mealy and spoil very quickly. Crunchy and tasty, the Asian pear, or nashi, is the latest pear to arrive in our fruit stores. Its shape often fools people into thinking it is a cross between an apple and a pear. This fruit will keep for up to two months in the fridge.

In the kitchen

Raw or cooked, pears can be used to make hors-d'oeuvres, salads and, of course, delicious desserts.

Recipes

☐ Pear compote (p. 136)
☐ Rice pudding with pear (p. 261)

Good to know

Canned pears contain almost none of the nutrients found in fresh pears. Moreover, they are usually soaking in high-calorie syrup.

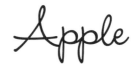

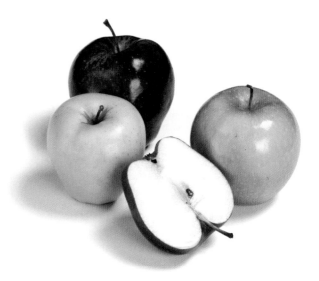

Succulent to bite into, excellent for your health, apples live up to their reputation. Besides being rich in vitamins and mineral salts, they contain an antioxidant substance called quercetin, which is capable of inhibiting the growth of cancer tumors and fighting inflammation. They also contain soluble and insoluble fiber, including pectin, that help lower cholesterol in the blood stream.

Other health benefits

◉ Helps prevent tooth decay
◉ Anti-diarrheal
◉ Lowers risk of cardiovascular disease
◉ Diuretic
◉ Laxative
◉ Energizing

Uses

The old proverb, "an apple a day keeps the doctor away", still rings true today, as long as you eat apples with the peel, where all its nutrients are stored. Eating an apple first thing every morning has an excellent purifying effect. Eating one at night before bedtime wards off constipation. Bite into an apple after a meal to clean your teeth, freshen your breath and tone your gums. Low in calories, it is the perfect snack for people trying to lose a few pounds.

Precautionary warning

Because they are sensitive to destructive insects, apples are often sprayed with pesticides throughout their growth. And to preserve them, they are coated with wax. If you can't buy organic apples, make sure to wash them thoroughly and eat them with the skin on.

Buying and storing

There exists a wide variety of apples; some of the best eating apples are: melba, gala, manintosh, red and yellow delicious, russet. Some of the best cooking apples (that can also be eaten raw) are: cortland, spartan, empire, idared, rome beauty. Generally, apples are picked before they're fully ripe and keep well in the fridge for many weeks.

In the kitchen

It is best to eat apples raw to preserve their properties. They are perfect to add to a fruit or vegetable salad. Cooked, they can be added to curries and stews. Of course, they always add amazing flavor when making compote, flan, fruit crisp and many other desserts.

Recipes

- Apple crisp with ginger (p. 266)
- Quick lentil and fruit picadillo with golden pita (p. 193)
- Sweet potato and apple mash (p. 240)

- Carrot and beet salad (p.165)
- Cabbage and apple salad (p. 183)
- Endive, fennel and apple salad (p. 169)

Good to know

Apple juice does not come close to a real apple in terms of health benefits. But it goes without saying that it is a much better choice than a soft drink.

Plum and prune

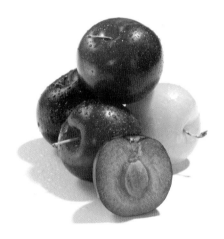

The plum is rich in potassium and vitamin A. It also contains an antioxidant that protects cells against the damaging effects of free radicals and diminishes certain signs of aging, such as joint pain. The prune is a plum that acquires iron, B vitamins and fiber in the dehydration process.

Other health benefits

- Hepatic decongestant
- Lowers cholesterol
- Energizing
- Relieves constipation

Precautionary warning

Can cause flatulence, nausea and other gastric discomfort if eaten in large quantities. To benefit fully from their properties, add them to your diet gradually.

Buying and storing

Choose a firm plum that has a smooth, shiny skin and store in the fridge. Prunes, like other dried fruit, should be kept in a dry, dark place.

In the kitchen

Eat prunes plain, add them to salads, or use them to make compote and jam. You can add prunes to rice, meat stews, desserts, fruit crisps or squares, and dried fruit compotes.

Recipe

- Rabbit with dried fruit (p. 226)

Good to know

Bottled prune juice has very little fiber, but is an excellent laxative.

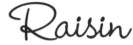

Raisin

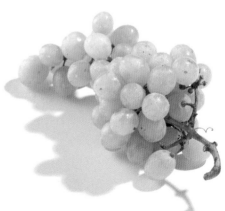

For as long as it has been harvested, the fruit of the vine has been greatly valued, not only for its therapeutic properties, but also for the incredible wine it produces. More recently, it has come to light that red wine is a powerful antioxidant that can lower the risk of heart conditions and cancer. Quercetin, the substance responsible for these effects, is also present in grapes, but it seems that the fermentation process required to make wine increases its powers. In the past few decades, researchers have examined the properties of flavonoids in grapes, especially resveratrol, which is mostly concentrated in the skin of the fruit, and oligo proanthocyanidin, which is found mainly in the seed envelope. Grapes are an excellent source of antioxidants and vitamin C; this makes them highly recommended for people who need to maintain healthy bones. Raisins have the same benefits as grapes, plus they contain other nutrients that are good for arthritis sufferers, such as mineral salts and B vitamins.

Other health benefits

- Lowers cholesterol
- Diminishes ocular stress brought on by glare
- Fights viruses

- Lowers risk of cardiovascular disease
- Laxative
- Prevents tooth decay
- Prevents skin aging
- Protects against different types of cancer
- Lowers high blood pressure
- Relieves hemorrhoids
- Tonic
- Treats vascular insufficiency and varicose veins

Uses

It is not advisable to overindulge in wine to get the benefits. The recommended daily intake is two glasses. Eating raisins regularly (6 to 8 grams per day) can lower cholesterol, improve intestinal function and lower the risk of colon cancer.

Precautionary warning

It is imperative to wash grapes thoroughly before eating, as their skin is contaminated with pollutants, pesticide residue, and mildew.

Buying and storing

Grapes keep well in the fridge, and they may even be frozen for a few days.

In the kitchen

Grapes are great raw, either to nibble on, or to add to a crudité or cheese platter, as well as fruit or vegetable salads. They go surprisingly well with venison in gravy. Raisins contain phyto-chemically-active tartaric acid. They can be used to make many different dishes, from entrées to desserts.

Recipes

- Kiwi compote with tea and ginger (p. 130)
- Rabbit with dried fruit (p. 226)
- Quick lentil and fruit picadillo with golden pita (p. 193)
- Cantaloupe and grape salad with ginger (p. 158)

Good to know

Red grapes contain twice as much phenolic compounds as green grapes making their anti-oxidant properties twice as powerful.

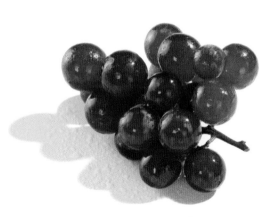

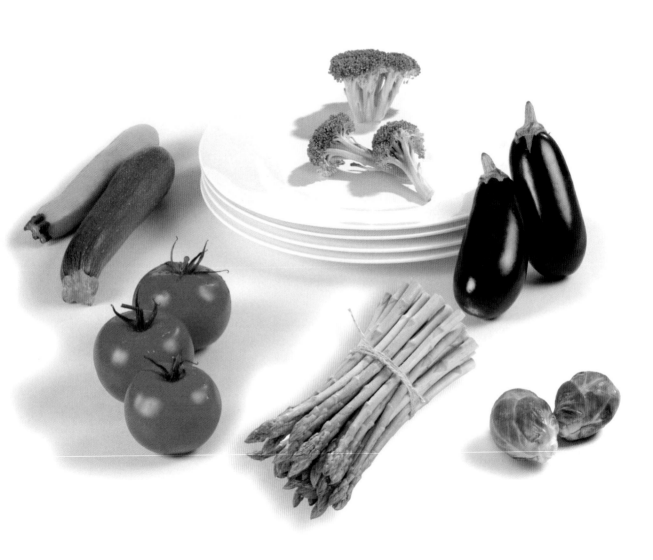

Vegetables

I've already described how I rediscovered the joy of eating fresh food. Since this dietary rebirth, my spouse and I have replaced our regular evening cocktail with a variety of fresh fruits and vegetables. This transition toward a healthier diet did not take place overnight. However, gradually, as we came to appreciate the naturally aperitif benefits that raw freshness provided, we traded our drinks for a plateful of crudités. We quickly noticed changes: we were more alert and felt less heavy after a meal, and we slept better. In my case, hip and back pain started to subside.

It's not rocket science: all you need to do is put together an appetizing plate full of varied raw vegetables – carrot sticks, celery ribs, strips of red or yellow sweet pepper, cauliflower and broccoli florets, cucumber and tomato slices, spinach leaves and other greens, to which we would add slices of melon, pieces of pear and apple, pineapple cubes and, in season, strawberries, raspberries and blueberries for beautiful contrasting colors. Bright color in food indicates the presence of health-friendly nutrients, but they also stimulate the appetite.

An entrée of raw food does not require much preparation and, alone, provides more than the daily recommended intake of fruits and vegetables, which is a minimum of five portions per day. Furthermore, because it is served first, the main meal can then be smaller. And all the antioxidants it offers will neutralize any fat contained in the foods eaten after.

I can't stress enough how this simple process is beneficial; not only is it healthy but it serves as a wonderful bonding ritual: the entire family can gather in the kitchen, washing, peeling, slicing and arranging these foods on the plate.

Another good way to incorporate raw vegetables in your diet is to serve them as snacks. If the idea of replacing your mid-day chocolate bar with broccoli does not appeal to you, try serving these miniature trees with dried fruit, apricots, strawberries, cranberries, grapes, almonds, or pistachios – the choices are endless. Just make sure your snack includes a good portion of vegetables; it's all in the presentation.

If you don't like raw vegetables, steam a few different kinds, just long enough to keep them crunchy, and then store them in an airtight container. They will keep three to four days in the fridge. You will have a ready-to-eat entrée when you get home from work. All you'll need to do is add a drizzle of oil and a dash of herbs. Again, lots of brightly-colored foods will be more enticing, so choose accordingly. Still unconvinced? Try some artichoke hearts and olives served with dried and fresh fruit. Always be careful not to choose foods that are high in calories or that are not recommended in your particular case. The idea is simply to increase your vegetable intake. After a few months of this new diet, you will notice improvements in your health and hopefully, feel less joint pain.

The best arthritis-fighting vegetables

Garlic

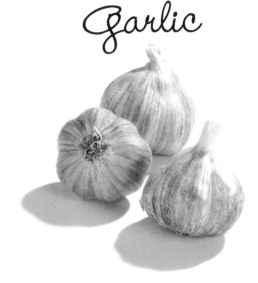

For centuries, humans all over the world have benefitted from the healing properties of this small and pungent bulb. Even though folk tradition is responsible for its title as king of plants, scientists today agree that its reputation is warranted and its therapeutic powers truly make it the king of the superfoods. Raw, it is an efficient antiviral agent. It is also an antioxidant, containing substances which prevent certain types of cancer, and reduce inflammation.

Other health benefits

- Antiseptic
- Promotes stomach function and stimulates appetite
- Lowers blood pressure and pulse rate
- Protects against cancer
- Tonic effect
- Anti-parasitic

Uses

It is recommended to eat two raw garlic cloves a day. To get all the antibacterial benefits, crush the cloves in a mortar, or with the blade of a knife, or chop finely. They can then be added to a salad with fresh lemon juice instead of vinegar. Crushing the garlic and adding lemon juice to it releases ajoene, an excellent anticoagulant compound.

Precautionary warning

Garlic powder does not provide any of garlic's health benefits. Garlic pills or capsules contain only traces of the active substances proprietary to fresh garlic. It is thought that the garlic germ is responsible for any digestive discomfort brought on by eating garlic. All you need to do is remove the green sprout hiding inside the clove. Consumed in large quantities, raw garlic can irritate sensitive stomachs and cause heartburn. Garlic is not recommended to people with dermatosis, eczema, bowel irritation or for lactating women. Garlic should not be eaten with sweet food or with milk. It doesn't react well with heated oil, fried foods and starches. If you want to benefit from garlic's healing properties, integrate it into your diet slowly and gradually, making sure you chew your food sufficiently. Cooked garlic loses its antiviral properties, but many others remain. It is a good idea to eat some every day, both cooked and raw. Garlic is a multi-beneficial ingredient that improves the flavor of many dishes.

Buying and storing

There are approximately 300 varieties of garlic. Common white garlic has the most medicinal and culinary properties. Choose firm bulbs that are plump and without sprouts. Brittle and dry bulbs indicate lack of freshness. Garlic will keep for many weeks in a dry, dark place with good air circulation.

In the kitchen

Garlic is one of the star ingredients in Mediterranean cooking. Gourmets and foodies the world over love the flavor and perfume it gives any dish. Other than in dessert, it can be added to most recipes and can be cooked in many ways.

Recipes

- Asian-style artichokes (p. 169)
- Duck en chemise with salted herbs (p. 223)
- Chickpea and vegetable curry, chicken alternative (p. 200)
- Poached turbot with fresh tomato (p. 213)
- Tarragon rabbit (p. 227)
- Short pasta with grilled vegetables (p. 194)
- Quick winter pesto (p. 251)
- Pizza with goat cheese and pesto (p. 178)
- Herb and garlic potatoes (p. 238)
- Kale soup (p. 142)
- Tomato and chickpea soup (p. 146)
- Basic tomato sauce (p. 250)
- Winter vegetable soup (p. 153)
- Spinach and white kidney bean soup (p. 150)

Good to know

The American National Cancer Institute lists garlic as the top cancer-fighting food.

Artichoke

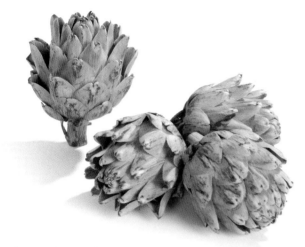

This edible burr was at one time reputed to be an aphrodisiac, but is now better known for its digestive benefits and blood-sugar lowering properties. It is low in fat and a good source of fiber, but higher in sodium than most other fruits and vegetables. It contains folic acid, a nutrient useful in bone formation, and magnesium and potassium, two minerals that play a role in the treatment of arthritis.

Other health benefits

- Energizing and stimulating
- Promotes urea and cholesterol elimination
- Relieves digestive problems
- Treats irritable bowel syndrome

Precautionary warning

Artichoke cooking water makes a good base for vegetable soup, but should be avoided in cases of gout, arthritis and urinary tract infections because of its high mineral concentration. Consumed in excess, it can cause intestinal discomfort and bloating. Artichoke leaf extract should not be used in cases of bile duct obstruction, because its bile-stimulating effects may cause serious problems.

Buying and storing

Choose a heavy, firm and compact artichoke with clean, closed leaves that are a nice olive green. A young artichoke will have tastier flesh. Discolored or rough open leaves indicate lack of freshness. Keep refrigerated in a plastic bag for up to one week.

In the kitchen

Always have canned artichoke hearts on hand. They are a quick, easy, and healthy food to serve, and are great on a crudités platter, or in a salad. If you prefer to eat them whole, they are quicker to prepare in the microwave than in a pot (see p. 169).

Recipes

- Asian-style artichokes (p. 169)
- Mini lasagna rolls with pistachios and artichoke hearts (p. 197)
- Winter tabbouleh with sun-dried tomato (p. 162)

Good to know

To eat an artichoke, peel the leaves off one at a time, starting at the outside. Suck the flesh off each one. As you eat your way to the heart, the leaves will become more succulent. The heart is the best part, but you have to remove the beard – or choke – before enjoying.

Asparagus

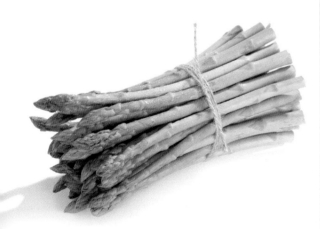

Few vegetable are as low in calories, while being as high in nutrients, as the asparagus. It contains many arthritis-friendly substances, such as carotene, vitamins C & E, and a finite amount of MSM, a sulfur compound that relieves joint pain.

Other health benefits

- Lowers cholesterol
- Purifying and diuretic
- Protects against cancer
- Protects against cardiovascular disease
- Remineralizes

Precautionary warning

Asparagus is not recommended for people with gout.

Buying and storage

Choose nice, green asparagus with smooth, firm, pointed, purplish tips. They can be frozen once blanched. Wrapped up tightly in foil and placed in an airtight container, they will keep in the freezer for up to a year.

In the kitchen

Served as an entrée or side dish, they are delicious with a vinaigrette. They are great served cold with a dip. To cook them, put them in a frying pan covered with cold water, bring to a boil and let simmer 3 to 5 minutes. Eat them right away or rinse them with cold water and store in the fridge for later use.

Recipe

 Asparagus with orange and pecans (p. 158)

Good to know

You might have noticed your urine has a distinct smell after eating asparagus. This is caused by methyl mercaptan, a harmless substance they contain.

Eggplant

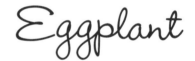

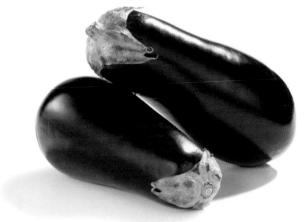

This beautiful vegetable with its voluptuous shape and deep, rich color is easy to digest and low in calories. It is also low in protein, carbohydrates and fats, but high enough in potassium that it has diuretic benefits. It is a good source of antioxidants, making it a good choice for arthritis sufferers.

Other health benefits

- Anti-anemic
- Helps to prevent cancer
- Diuretic
- Lowers cholesterol
- Stimulates the liver and pancreas

Uses

It is recommended to eat this vegetable at least once a week, keeping in mind that it also fights age-related diseases.

Precautionary warning

Even thought eggplant is low in calories, is has the ability to absorb great amounts of fat when fried, so it is best to eat it raw in hors-d'oeuvres or cooked in stews and sauces.

Buying and storing

The skin should be deep purple and smooth to the touch with a prickly, dark green stem. It will keep for many days in the fridge. It will get wrinkly as it dries out and no longer be edible. An eggplant is ripe when your fingers leave a slight imprint on its skin.

In the kitchen

Many countries use eggplant to make tasty traditional specialty dishes: moussaka (Greece – see p. 201), ratatouille (France), baba ganoush (Lebanon), eggplant parmagiana (Italy). It gives unique flavor to tomato sauce.

Recipes

- Lentil moussaka (p. 201)
- Short pasta with grilled vegetables (p. 194)
- Layered chicken and eggplant (p. 220)

Good to know

A younger eggplant's flesh will be more tender and less bitter. Choose a longer-shaped eggplant; it will contain fewer seeds, which give it its bitterness.

Beets

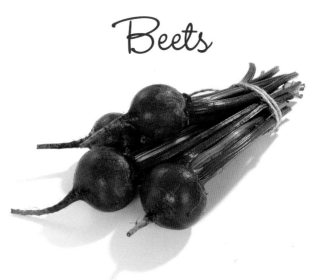

The entire beet is edible, including the stems and leaves (otherwise known as beet greens), but its root is the most popular. It is rich in potassium and iron, and is a good source of folic acid. The juice is reputed to relieve arthritis symptoms.

Other health benefits

- Fights anemia
- Highly digestible
- Energizing and nutritious
- Prevents congenital malformations
- Protects against cardiovascular disease and certain cancers
- Relieves constipation

Home remedy

To treat flu and anemia, drink a small glass of beet juice every day for one month.

Precautionary warning

Beets are not recommended for diabetics.

Buying and storing

It is best to buy small or medium-sized beets that will be easier to peel once cooked.

In the kitchen

It is recommended to eat beets raw to get more of their nutrients. If you prefer to eat them cooked, it is best to leave them unpeeled to preserve their nutrients: boil them or bake them wrapped in parchment paper.

Recipes

☐ Beets infused with orange (microwave) (p. 234)
☐ Quick beet and carrot salad (p. 165)

Broccoli

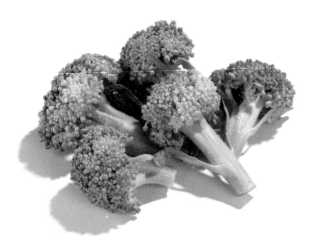

B roccoli is rich in vitamin C - one of the vegetables with the highest content - and beta-carotene, two substances that make it a powerful antioxidant. It also has a high fiber concentration.

Other health benefits

◉ Lowers risk of cancer
◉ Protects against cardiovascular disease

Home remedy

Eat a bouquet of broccoli florets every day to ward off arthritis symptoms.

Precautionary warning

There are no known contra-indications for this excellent superfood.

Buying and storing

Look for firm, dark green stems with small, compact florets, dark green or purplish in color. Disregard any that have soft stems and yellowing florets, indicating a lack of freshness. Stored in the fridge, wrapped in perforated plastic, broccoli will keep for a week.

In the kitchen

Broccoli makes a great soup cooked in broth with zucchini and onions. Steam it or cook it in a pressure cooker to accompany grilled meat and fish or use it in a casserole. Served raw, it adds crunch to salads and its pretty florets decorate your crudités platter.

Recipe

☐ Broccoli soup (p. 152)

Good to know

Broccoli only loses a small amount of its vitamins when cooked, except when microwaved, where it will lose most of its nutrients. That said, it is always best to eat it raw.

Carrot

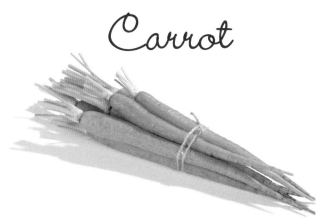

Carrots are an excellent source of beta-carotene, pectin, potassium and fiber. It is one of the vegetables with the most medicinal properties. Its rejuvenating juice is good for the liver and is highly recommended to arthritis sufferers.

Other health benefits

- Anti-anemic
- Improves night vision
- Fights bacterial infections
- Lowers cholesterol
- Remineralizes
- Strengthens the immune system
- Relieves constipation
- Relieves diarrhea

Uses

Eating one raw carrot a day is like taking a natural medication brimming with benefits. We know that people who eat carrots every day are less likely to develop macular degeneration and cardiovascular disease.

Precautionary warning

It is better to leave carrots unpeeled to enjoy all their benefits. Buy organic carrots – they haven't been treated – or scrub and scrape under cold running water.

Buying and storing

Carrots sold with their greens – or tops— taste better, but all carrots keep for many weeks in the fridge.

In the kitchen

There are hundreds of ways to use carrots. They can be used in soups, entrées, or side dishes and make excellent cakes, cookies and muffins. Carrot juice is delicious and full of nutrients. Carrot tops make good soup and can be added to salads and sauces.

Recipes

- Chickpea and vegetable curry (p. 200)
- Tortilla cups with curry chicken (p. 179)
- Carrot cake (p. 265)
- Grilled honey-glazed vegetables (p. 237)
- Root vegetables en chemise (p. 237)
- Carrot and ginger soup (p. 142)
- Parsnip, carrot and sweet potato purée (p. 240)
- Carrot and beet salad (p. 165)
- Salade de chou et de pommes (p. 183)
- Cabbage and apple salad (p. 183)
- Clementine and orange salad with sage (p. 160)
- Quick fish soup (p. 149)
- Quick minestrone (p. 148)

Good to know

Carrots do not lose their medicinal properties when cooked. Eating lots of carrots can cause the skin to turn yellowish, but this is not harmful and skin color will go back to normal if carrot consumption is reduced to a reasonable quantity.

Celery

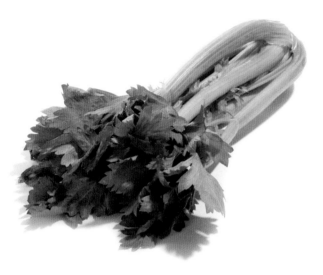

Celery is low in calories, rich in fiber and made up of 95% water. Its leaves contain vitamins A & C, calcium, iron and potassium. Its high content of complex compounds may, according to recent studies, stop tumor cell growth. Its juice. applied directly to a wound, will promote healing. Celery seeds contain a substance that helps fight cancer, among many other medicinal properties. They are recommended in the treatment of flu, insomnia, indigestion, as well as arthritis. Low in calories, celery is a perfect appetite-suppressant snack for anyone watching their weight.

Other health benefits
- Lowers blood pressure
- Digestive and astringent

Home remedy
People with rheumatism should drink half a glass of celery juice every day for 15 days.

Precautionary warning
Even though celery helps fight hypertension, celery leaves and celery salt are not recommended for people on a low-sodium diet because of their high-sodium content.

Buying and storing
Make sure the stalks and leaves are firm and fresh. Celery keeps for many days in the fridge, wrapped in perforated plastic. If it softens, you can crisp it up by soaking it in cold water and then refrigerating for a few hours.

In the kitchen
Celery is usually enjoyed raw, but it gives lots of good flavor to soups, sauces and stews. Don't discard the leaves, as they are packed with flavor – perfect for any broth or soup. The seeds are also very flavorful and can be used in stuffing and with poached vegetables.

Recipes
- Home-made vegetable broth (p. 144)
- Celery soup with turmeric (p. 150)
- Chicken salad with chickpeas (p. 184)
- Quick minestrone (p. 148)

Good to know
Celery does not lose its nutritional value in cooking. On the other hand, soaking it will cause it to lose some nutrients.

Celeriac

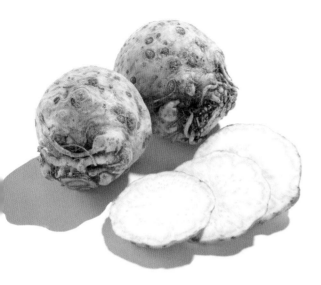

Buying and storing
Look for a firm, unblemished root. It will keep over a week in the fridge. Celeriac is also available canned.

In the kitchen
It is more popular in Europe, where it is often served on a crudités platter, than in America. It is delicious cooked in soups, purées and casseroles. It is delicious raw in a salad or plain, drizzled with vinaigrette.

Good to know
It is the vegetable with the most sodium.

L ike its stalky cousin, celeriac is a root vegetable rich in fiber, potassium and vitamin C. There is, however, no physical family resemblance, as its shape is more like a rutabaga than celery. Its flavor is also quite different— sharper and stronger-tasting. It keeps well, making it a perfect winter vegetable.

Other health benefits
- Antiseptic
- Refreshing
- Digestive and tonic
- Stimulates the adrenal glands

Uses
Eat twice a week raw, grated, or in fine strips to improve digestion.

Precautionary warning
Like celery, celeriac is rich in sodium, and therefore not recommended for low-salt diets.

Cabbage

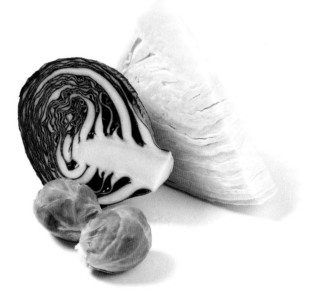

U ninspiring to look at but available all year long, green cabbage is packed with vitamins, minerals and antibacterial substances. The list of conditions treated by cabbage, internally and externally, over the centuries is so long it seems ridiculous. But respectable historians claim that the Romans considered it a panacea and used it for hundreds of years to stay healthy and treat all sorts of maladies. Due to its high carotene content, it is useful in preventing age-related conditions, such as cataracts and joint degeneration.

Other health benefits

- Promotes healing
- Kills viruses
- Lowers cancer risk, especially breast, colon, prostate and stomach cancers
- Promotes growth
- Heals ulcers and varicose veins
- Prevents colds
- Relieves shingles

Home remedy

Flatten a cabbage leaf with a rolling pin and apply directly on a painful joint. Keep this compress on for 30 minutes to two hours.

Uses

Eating raw cabbage at least three times a week offers surprisingly undeniable protection against many afflictions.

Precautionary warning

Whether raw or steamed, cabbage is easy to digest. But in order to retain all of its extraordinary properties, it is best to avoid cooking in water.

Buying and storing

Look for a heavy cabbage with firm, green leaves that have no marks or tears. It will last up to a month, kept in the fridge in a plastic bag. Savoy cabbage has dark green, curly leaves that keep their curl when cooked. Bok choy is a favorite in Asia; it has large, green leaves and white stalks that resemble celery ribs. Kale, or curly kale, tastes a lot like rapini and is prepared much like spinach.

In the kitchen

Napa cabbage, or Chinese cabbage, has a more delicate taste. Bok choy, a green Chinese vegetable, is mostly served cooked. Red cabbage, white cabbage, Milan cabbage and Brussels sprouts all have more or less the same properties as green cabbage. Forget the ever-present soggy coleslaw and discover the true flavor of raw cabbage. Sliced finely and tossed in a fresh salad with a drizzle of olive oil and lemon juice, its flavor comes to life. Combined with your favorite fruits and vegetables - apple, pear, clementine - it makes a refreshing and appetizing entrée. Pair cabbage with carrot for a powerful, antioxidant dynamic duo. Choose a young cabbage, and remove the outer, tougher leaves and the hard stem before preparing. Cabbage is a pure delight when served as an entrée with a light vinaigrette accompanying a salad of fresh greens, cubed pear and almonds. Cook bok choy leaves like spinach and its ribs like you would cook celery.

Recipes

- Kale soup (p. 142)
- Winter vegetable soup (p. 153)
- Cabbage and apple salad (p. 183)
- Red cabbage salad (p. 165)
- Salmon pasta salad (p. 180)

Good to know

Attention sauerkraut lovers, this dish should be avoided in cases of hypertension, but it is not as bad as formerly thought, as long as it is prepared following a natural process. The worst thing about it is the salted meats that are often added in excess.

Cauliflower

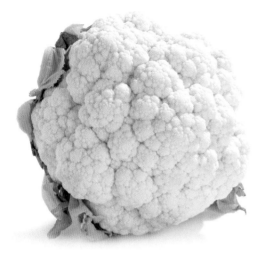

Like all members of the cruciferous family, cauliflower is rich in fiber, phosphorus, potassium and vitamin C, four nutrients that help in treating arthritis.

Other health benefits

- Prevents colds and flu
- Protects against cancer, especially breast, colon and prostate cancers

Uses

A 100-gram serving of raw cauliflower a day provides the daily recommended intake of vitamin C.

Precautionary warning

People suffering from gout should avoid cauliflower and choose cabbage or broccoli, because these contain fewer amino acids. The puric acid in cauliflower can trigger a painful gout attack. Cauliflower can also cause flatulence when the bowel breaks down its cellulose content. For this reason, you should add it to your diet gradually.

Buying and storing

Choose a heavy vegetable with green leaves and lovely cream-colored florets. Brown markings indicate lack of freshness. Do not wash until ready to use, wrap in perforated plastic and store in the fridge where it will keep for a week.

In the kitchen

Cooked in broth alone, or with carrots or broccoli, cauliflower makes a tasty soup with great texture. The crunch of its florets is a welcome addition to any salad or crudités platter. Cauliflower is an excellent appetite suppressant.

Recipes

- Fusilli with cauliflower and cherry tomatoes (p. 190)
- Creamy cauliflower soup (p. 146)

Good to know

The cauliflower is the easiest member of the cabbage family to digest.

Summer squash

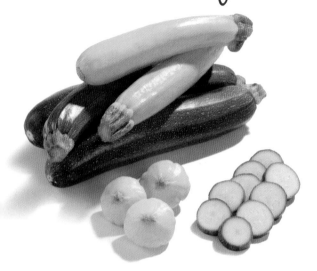

Good to know

The cocozelle zucchini is similar to its cousin, but larger, with stripes and a mild flavor. It can also be stuffed and baked.

Zucchini is certainly the most popular of all summer squash, but the round and flat pattypan squash and the pear-shaped chayote are other varieties worth discovering. All these squash have a delicate taste, are easy to digest and are good sources of fiber and vitamins A & C.

Other health benefits
⊛ Protects against different types of cancer

Uses
Adding unpeeled squash to a meat dish improves digestion.

Buying and storing
Choose heavy zucchini with nice, green skin; pattypans should be free of blemishes; and chayotes should be firm and smooth. They all keep well in the fridge.

In the kitchen
Zucchini is used in all sorts of dishes: soups, entrées, casseroles, salads, cakes and muffins. The chayote is almost as versatile, except when it comes to desserts. Pattypan squash are usually served stuffed.

Winter squash

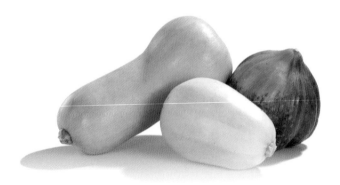

There are many kinds of winter squash, some of them are: the caramel-colored and bell-shaped butternut squash; the bright orange and green knobby Hubbard squash; the yellow oval-shaped spaghetti squash; and every kid's favorite, the pumpkin. The butternut and the Hubbard squash both have more than the daily recommended requirement of beta-carotene. The pumpkin is also rich in beta-carotene, while its seeds (see p. 115) contain the most valuable nutrients for fighting arthritis.

Other health benefits
- Lowers the risk of endometrial cancer
- Prevents heart conditions
- Prevents lung conditions
- Relieves constipation
- Relieves hemorrhoids

Precautionary warning
There are no ill-effects associated with winter squash; they can be consumed safely.

Buying and storing
Look for heavy gourds with hard skin; they will keep for many weeks, or all winter, in a cool, dry place at a temperature of 53 oF Choosing a squash that still has its stem ensures that the inside will still be good.

In the kitchen
Butternut squash is delicious mashed with carrot and rutabaga. Hubbard and acorn squash are very good halved, stuffed with rice, and baked in the oven (see p. 176) or served with a meat hash. Add pieces of hubbard to a stew to increase its vitamin content. Pumpkin makes amazing soups and desserts.

Recipes
- Squash and fennel soup (p. 152)
- Squash stuffed with salmon and rice (p. 176)

Good to know
A darker color indicates a squash with a higher beta-carotene content.

Watercress

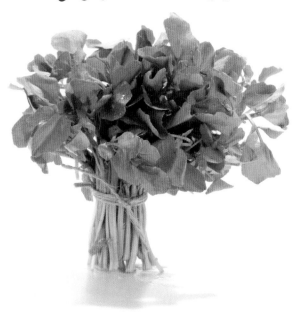

Celebrated for centuries for its healing properties, watercress is a medicinal herb that is used to treat scurvy—in fact, it was called scurvy grass. Today, scurvy is not very common, but watercress is rich in vitamin C (almost as much as a lemon), making it an ideal food for arthritis sufferers.

Other health benefits
- Anti-anemic
- Antidote to nicotine
- Purifying
- Diuretic
- Protects against cardiovascular disease

Uses
Use watercress in place of lettuce in sandwiches and salads, to benefit from extra protection against disease. Smokers should eat watercress daily; it has been proven to protect against lung cancer.

Precautionary warning

Eating too much watercress can irritate sensitive stomachs or trigger the symptoms of cystitis (inflammation of the bladder).

Buying and storing

Choose a bunch with nice, green leaves and put it in a plastic bag before storing it in the fridge. You can also place it in a glass of water wrapped in plastic before putting it in the fridge. It will keep no longer than four to five days.

In the kitchen

Watercress can be cooked, but it will lose many of its therapeutic properties. Added raw to salads and used to garnish crudités, it is a veritable bouquet of vitamins.

Recipe

☐ Mango and watercress salad (p. 170)

Good to know

One ½-cup serving of watercress contains more vitamin C than the daily recommended intake.

Spinach

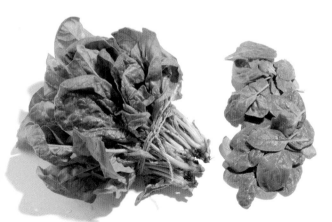

These lovely green leaves store an important source of fiber, vitamins C & E, and chlorophyll, as well as useful mineral salts. But its richness in carotenoids and beta-carotene are what make it a superfood for arthritis sufferers. Studies have shown that people who eat spinach regularly are less at risk for certain cancers, especially lung cancer. Spinach has also surpassed the green bean as the vegetable of choice for weight loss.

Other health benefits

- Activates pancreatic secretions
- Anti-anemic
- Promotes good eye sight
- Fights depression
- Protects against different types of cancer
- Lowers cholesterol
- Regulates intestinal function
- Cardiotonic

Uses

Eating fresh spinach and similar leafy vegetables twice a week offers valuable protection against disease and regulates mood.

Precautionary warning

Cooked spinach does not keep well because it encourages nitrite proliferation. Some people are sensitive to spinach and risk urinary calculus. Their high content of oxalic acid interferes with calcium absorption, but you would have to eat a lot of spinach for this to be a problem.

Buying and storing

Look for nice, green leaves as young as possible. They will keep five to six weeks refrigerated in a perforated plastic bag.

In the kitchen

Combine raw spinach leaves with lettuce for a fresh and healthy salad. Cook them in soups, stews, casseroles and puff pastry. Spinach is delicious with meat.

Recipes

- Cantaloupe and grape salad with ginger (p. 158)
- Spinach and white kidney bean soup (p. 150)

Good to know

Recent studies concluded that despite its long-standing reputation as an iron powerhouse, spinach, in fact, has 10 times less iron than was originally thought. A simple math error is at the heart of this misconception: when evaluating the iron content, apparently the experts' calculations were off a decimal.

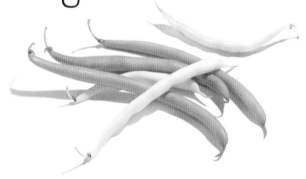

Green and yellow beans

Both green and yellow beans offer excellent nutritional properties. Low in fat and sodium, rich in vitamins, they satisfy a good part of the daily requirement of vitamin C. Green beans contain quercetin, a powerful antioxidant, and are a good source of silicium, which is beneficial to bone health.

Other health benefits

- Contribute to fetal development
- Fight infections
- Restorative
- Stimulate the liver and pancreas

Anti-anemia treatment

Add them to your menu two or three times a week to facilitate digestion and provide essential nutrients.

Precautionary warning

It is best to not overcook fresh beans and to eat them *al dente* to preserve all of their therapeutic properties.

Buying and storing

Look for unpackaged green and yellow beans so you can pick the best ones. Choose beans with a nice, bright color, avoiding the wrinkly, dried out, soft and discolored ones. Thin beans are more tender. To freeze, blanch for 3 minutes and keep no longer than one month.

In the kitchen

Fresh beans are an excellent vegetable side dish and add flavor to soups and salads. They can be boiled, steamed or microwaved.

Recipe

- Green beans with lemon and almonds (p. 236)

Good to know

Green beans are easy to grow in a plant pot or in your vegetable garden.

Dried beans and legumes

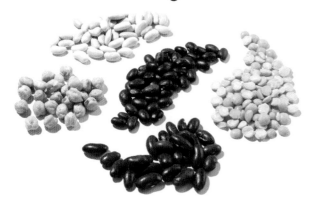

The white, red and green kidney beans, the Pinto bean, the chickpea, the black bean, the black gram and the lentil are some of the better known legumes. Once referred to as "the meat of the poor," they are the plant food that contains the most protein and they are rich in fiber. They protect against cardiovascular disease and may prevent certain cancers.

Other health benefits

- Lower cholesterol
- Contribute to fetal development
- Energizing and nutritious
- Prevent cardiovascular disease
- Regenerate nervous system

Health maintenance

Eat legumes two or three times a week to load up on fiber and protect against free radicals.

Precautionary warning

Dried beans cause flatulence. To prevent this, refer to the chart below, ensuring that beans are soaked long enough in frequent water changes, cook them sufficiently in fresh water and chew adequately.

Buying and storing

Dried beans keep for long periods of time if stored in airtight containers. They are widely available canned, which does not harm their nutritional properties.

In the kitchen

Dried beans can be used in a wide range of dishes: entrées, dips, vegetable salads, pasta salads, pâtés, stews and delicious soups. Before cooking them, they need to be rehydrated by soaking them for four to six hours, or overnight. Cook them in boiling water after rinsing them. Cooking time varies between one to two hours, depending on the kind of beans used and their age. Lentils do not require soaking but must be rinsed first. Red lentils, being smaller, are ideal in soups; green and brown lentils make delicious salads.

Cooking table

Legumes*	Soaking	Cooking time
Red kidney bean (and white or black)	6 hours	90 minutes
Soy bean	6 hours	3 hours
Red lentil	none	30 minutes
Green lentil	none	50 minutes
Split pea	none	50 minutes
Chickpea	6 hours	3 hours

For more on soy beans, see page 81.

*   *1 cup of dried beans yields 2 cups of cooked beans.*

Recipes

Good to know

Canned legumes do not lose their nutritional value and help make quick and easy meals. They can replace potatoes in soups and stews. They are also an excellent meat-substitute for any vegetarian diet.

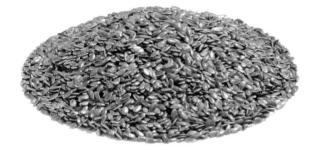

Flax (seed)

Flax has a fascinating story. For centuries, it has been used in many different ways – in textiles, canvas and paint. More recently, it has been added to cattle feed after observing that it was amazingly beneficial to human health. Flaxseed is a source of alpha-linolenic acid, a type of omega-3 fatty acid. It was first cultivated on the American continent by some of the first farmers to come from Europe.

Other health benefits

- Lowers bad cholesterol (LDL)
- Increases good cholesterol (HDL)
- Improves mood
- Lowers risk of cardiovascular disease
- Contributes to renal function
- Prevents breast, uterine, colon and prostate cancers
- Prevents osteoporosis in postmenopausal women

Uses

It is recommended to add two to three tablespoons of ground flaxseed to cereal, yogurt or salad every day to fully benefit from this plant's medicinal properties.

Precautionary warning

To obtain maximum benefits, seeds must be ground, as the body cannot break down their hard shell. It would seem that cooking cancels out their healthy effects. Whole flaxseed is not recommended for people suffering from diverticulitis, because they can get lodged in the lining of the intestine and cause inflammation.

Buying and storing

Buy whole flaxseed that will keep well in an airtight container in the freezer.

In the kitchen

Beware of recipes that add flaxseed to flour to make cakes, breads and muffins because their properties will vanish in baking. However, it is easy to incorporate flaxseed into your diet by adding ground flaxseed to breakfast cereal, juice, yogurt and smoothies. It is also possible to make the seed germinate and add the sprouts to salads.

Recipe

☐ Chickpea patty (p. 182)

Good to know

Flaxseed is richer in omega-3s than avocado and cold-water fish, even though these are good sources of alpha-linolenic acid. Many major egg producers have added flaxseed to their chicken feed, introducing omega-3 fatty acid-enriched eggs to the market.

Onion

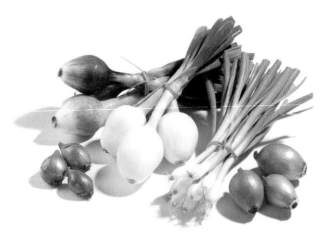

For centuries, the onion has been respected as a food with healing properties often considered miraculous. Even today, this tear-inducing bulb is valued for its therapeutic powers in healing infections and promoting health. Like its cousin garlic, it is a powerful, natural antibiotic. Rich in vitamin C, it contains numerous minerals and trace elements that offer antioxidant and immune system protection, while being low in calories.

Other health benefits

- Lowers blood sugar levels
- Lowers bad cholesterol (LDL)
- Increases and stimulates good cholesterol (HDL)
- Stimulates appetite
- Bronchial decongestant
- Treats respiratory problems
- Kills bacteria
- Reduces inflammation
- Promotes hair growth
- Clarifies blood
- Stops cancer cell growth
- Prevents atherosclerosis
- Slows down coagulation
- Stabilizes blood sugar

Uses

It is recommended to eat onions daily. One example of the onion's power: one half onion can increase HDL cholesterol levels by 30%. One tablespoon of cooked onion eaten after a meal rich in fat will stop the blood from thickening. Like many vegetables, its properties are strongest when eaten raw.

Home remedy

Rheumatism-fighting decoction

Drink one glass of this beverage first thing in the morning and one glass at bedtime: take 3 onions, cut but unpeeled, and boil for 15 minutes in 4 cups of water. Strain and store in the fridge.

Precautionary warning

Onions have very few known ill-effects, but may cause migraines for some people.

Buying and storing

Many varieties of onion are available, such as: sweet, red, white, and yellow onions. Look for onions that have not sprouted. They will keep for many weeks in a dark, dry place.

In the kitchen

Onion and all its family members (shallot, Welsh onion, chive, garlic, green onion, etc.), give as much flavor as nutritional value to a multitude of dishes. The green onion is an immature yellow onion. Dried chives have a more delicate flavor. Without these wonderful bulbs, it is hard to imagine what broths, soups, salads, marinades, vinaigrettes, pâtés, purees, meatloaves, casseroles, stews and sauces would taste like.

Recipes

- Poached turbot with fresh tomatoes (p. 213)
- Tarragon rabbit (p. 227)
- Pizza with goat cheese and pesto (p. 178)
- Fresh tomato pizza (p. 184)
- Green pea soup (p. 144)
- Black bean salad (p. 162)
- Spaghetti with zucchini and hazelnuts (p. 194)
- Chicken and chickpea salad (p. 184)
- Winter vegetable soup (p. 153)

Good to know

Approximately 44 million tons of onions are produced yearly all over the world, ranking it the second most-produced vegetable after the tomato. Greek scientists have recently discovered that onions lose a good part of their anti-oxidant properties when cooked. Shallots have unique properties. One tablespoon of chopped shallot contains a megadose of vitamin A that can strengthen the immune system and protect vision from age-related problems, such as cataracts and night blindness.

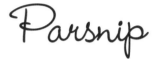

Parsnip

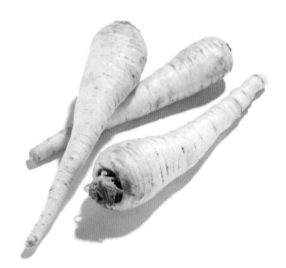

Related to the carrot and to parsley, this unassuming and slightly sweet root vegetable offers many benefits. It is low in calories and very nutritious, containing vitamin C, mineral salts and insoluble fiber – a perfect food for arthritis sufferers.

Other health benefits

- Improves mood
- Lowers risk of colon cancer
- Promotes digestion
- Protects against congenital malformations

Uses

A soup made with parsnip, leek and onion is a good way to benefit from the many properties all of these vegetables offer to boost health and fight cancer.

Precautionary warning

Excessive consumption of parsnip – somewhat unlikely du to its relative unpopularity – can cause skin to become light-sensitive because of its high coumarin content.

Buying and storing

Choose smooth, firm and unblemished roots that are not too big or they will be fibrous. Cut the stems and tops off and put them in a perforated plastic bag; they will keep approximately two weeks in the fridge.

In the kitchen

Much like the carrot, the parsnip adds crunch to crudités, is delicious pureed and is good in soups and stews. It is lovely grated raw in a salad. Cooked, it goes very well with other root vegetables. It is recommended to peel it after cooking to preserve its health properties.

Recipes

☐ Chickpea and vegetable curry (p. 200)
☐ Honey-glazed roasted vegetables (p. 237)
☐ Root vegetables en chemise (p. 237)
☐ Mashed parsnip, carrot and sweet potato (p. 240)
☐ Quick minestrone (p. 148)

Good to know

One 150-gram portion of parsnip contains 400 mg of potassium or, 16% of the recommended daily requirement.

Sweet potato

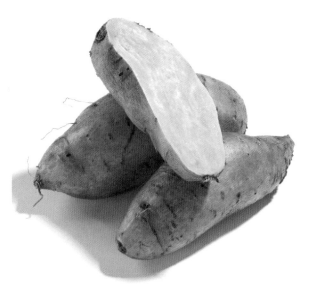

This tuberous root is only distantly related to the potato and totally unrelated to yams. The sweet potato is rich in vitamins A, B6, C & E, as well as in mineral salts and beta-carotene, which makes it extremely beneficial to arthritis sufferers. It offers good protection against cardiovascular disease and different types of cancer. It is low in calories and quite filling, making it a food of choice for diabetics and people watching their weight.

Other health benefits

- Lowers blood sugar levels
- Helps to improve memory
- Lowers cancer risk
- Detoxifies
- Stimulates the brain

Uses

Because of its many beneficial properties, the sweet potato is a better choice than the ordinary potato and is delicious with meat and fish dishes.

Precautionary warning

Beta-carotene needs fat to break through the intestinal wall; it is therefore recommended to eat sweet potato with a bit of fat to benefit from its protective qualities.

Buying and storing

Look for orange-colored tubers; as for all beta-carotene vegetables, it should have a deep, bright color. Firm and smooth, devoid of spots and blemishes, the sweet potato does not like to be stored in the fridge but will keep for a month in a cool (between 44 and 57 °C) and dark place.

In the kitchen

The sweet potato is cooked much like a potato, but with a shorter cooking time. It can be boiled, fried, pureed or used in salads, soups and stews. It also goes well in cakes and desserts because of its sweetness.

Recipes

☐ Sweet potato and apple mash (p. 240)
☐ Mashed parsnip, carrot and sweet potato (p. 240)

Good to know

One 115-gram portion of sweet potato contains 28 mg of vitamin C, or half of the daily recommended intake.

Leek

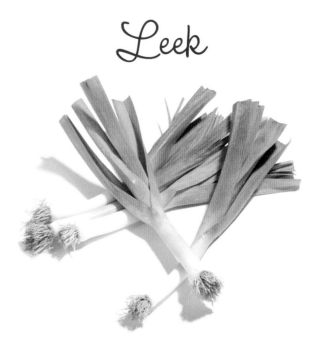

Like its relatives, onion and garlic, the leek is also rich in mineral salts and shares many of its relatives' beneficial properties, with the added bonus of a high folic acid content. Low in sodium and calories, it is rich in provitamin A and vitamins C & E for cellular antioxidant protection.

Other health benefits

⚬ Kills bacteria
⚬ Diuretic and astringent
⚬ Protects against cardiovascular disease

Uses

With its mild and delicate taste, it will appeal to those not so fond of onion, who will also profit from its benefits.

Precautionary warning

Leeks may cause flatulence because of the sulfur they contain. Furthermore, they should be thoroughly washed to remove all the soil and sand that gets stuck in the leaves.

Buying and storing

Choose a firm leek with nice, green leaves. Do not buy any that don't have their roots: they will spoil faster. Leeks keep well in the fridge.

In the kitchen

Raw leek will give salads a delicate taste. Cooked leek is delicious in soups, casseroles, quiches and rice; it is often served braised as a side-dish.

Recipes

- Honey-glazed roasted vegetables (p. 237)
- Creamy cauliflower soup (p. 146)
- Celery soup with turmeric (p. 150)
- Squash and fennel soup (p. 152)
- Cold cucumber soup (p. 149)
- Spicy rice with peppers (p. 241)

Good to know

One serving of cooked leek contains almost a third of the daily intake of folic acid recommended for adults.

Green pea

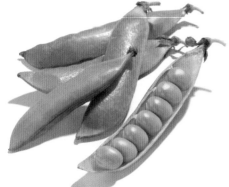

A pod-vegetable, the green pea is rich in mineral salts and vitamins as well as lutein, a complex substance that gives it its color and slows down the aging process. The snow pea also shares these properties, which are helpful in keeping joints flexible.

Other health benefits

- Lowers LDL cholesterol
- Energizing
- Promotes bowel evacuation
- Protects against cancer
- Prevents cataracts
- Relieves cold symptoms

Precautionary warning

Because they are very good at flushing out the bowel, peas are not recommended for people suffering from enteritis (intestinal inflammation).

Buying and storing

Fresh green peas are only available for a short time, but no need to worry: frozen peas offer the same nutritional properties.

In the kitchen

Green peas can be used in soups and stews, and they often accompany meat and fish.

Recipe

- Green pea soup (p. 144)

Good to know

Although scientists haven't quite figured out the amount of peas one would have to eat to benefit from the cancer-fighting chlorophyllin they contain, it is nonetheless recommended to include them in your diet as often as possible, along with other dark green vegetables. Canned green peas lose a good many nutrients in the canning process, but retain their lutein, which slows down the aging process and prevents cataracts.

Frozen peas retain most of their nutrients, including vitamin C.

Sweet pepper

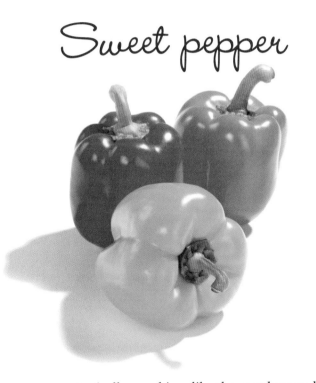

Botanically-speaking, like the eggplant and the tomato, the sweet pepper is a fruit. Whether red, orange or yellow, it is rich in beta-carotene and flavonoids, both of which bolster the effects of the vitamin C essential to arthritis sufferers. It also contains mineral salts and B vitamins. Because of the tag-team effect associated with vitamin C and beta-carotene in preventing signs of aging, elderly arthritis sufferers have much to gain by adding sweet peppers to their diet.

Other health benefits
- Protects the immune system
- Lowers risk of cardiovascular disease

Uses
Raw sweet pepper added twice weekly to salads will strengthen the immune system and protect against infections.

Precautionary warning
Sweet green peppers at full size have not reach full maturity and can be difficult to digest. The antioxidant vitamin C contained in sweet peppers is not resistant to cooking; it is best to eat them raw.

Buying and storing
Sweet peppers are available in a rainbow of colors: yellow, orange, red, green and even purple. They all keep well in the fridge.

In the kitchen
Left raw, they add a nice crunch to salads; cooked, they add nice flavor to soups, rice and stews.

Recipes
- Black bean burrito (p. 180)
- Chickpea and vegetable curry (p. 200)
- Tortilla cup with chicken and curry (p. 179)
- Pasta with sweet pepper coulis (p. 196)
- Short pasta with roasted vegetables (p. 194)
- Fresh tomato pizza (p. 184)
- Spicy rice with sweet peppers (p. 241)
- Black bean salad (p. 162)
- Chicken and chickpea salad (p. 184)
- Endive and fennel salad with apple (p. 250)

Good to know
A sweet red pepper contains more vitamin C than an orange of the same weight. The riper the sweet pepper, the deeper the color and the richer in nutrients. Red sweet pepper contains nine times the carotenoids of sweet green pepper.

Potato

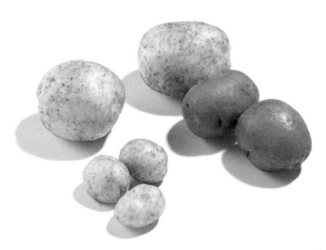

The potato has been perceived many different ways since its discovery in Chili in the 16th century. When it was first introduced in France, it was considered harmful to the health. Whether praised for its rheumatism- and virus-fighting properties, or rejected by scientists for its supposed lack of nutritional value, the potato still remains one of the most popular, as well as controversial, vegetables. It is rich in potassium, which helps lower blood pressure, and its vitamin B content makes it good for arthritis sufferers. Furthermore, its skin contains complex substances that can absorb cancer-causing agents in smoked foods such as barbecued meat.

Other health benefits
- Lowers blood pressure
- Relieves ulcer discomfort

Uses
Unfortunately, it is the unpeeled, raw potato that is healthiest, a fact that might disappoint many. However, oven-baking gives it good flavor, and preserves most of its properties. It remains low in calories as long as no fat is added, so it can be eaten often this way, just mind the butter and the sour cream!

Precautionary warning
Experts do not all agree on this point, but the potato is generally not recommended for diabetics, as it elevates glycemia. Germinating or green-tinged potatoes contain solanines, a substance that can be toxic in sufficient quantities. Never bake a potato that has germinated, or eat its skin.

Buying and storing
There are varieties of potato that suit every type of cooking (oven-baked, deep-fried, mashed or pan-fried), they are: russet, Idaho and Yukon Gold. New potatoes are excellent boiled and make a great salad. Look for potatoes with nice skin, free of sprouts. Store them in a cool place, but not in the fridge. Do not store them with onions; they will absorb the potatoes' moisture and make them decompose faster.

In the kitchen
There are many ways to prepare potatoes and they are a welcome addition to many dishes, such as salads, soups, stews and casseroles.

Recipes
- Oven-fried potatoes (p. 236)
- Honey-glazed roasted vegetables (p. 237)
- Meatless shepherd's pie (p. 192)
- Herb and garlic potatoes (p. 238)

Good to know
The yellower the flesh, the higher the vitamin C concentration.

Soy

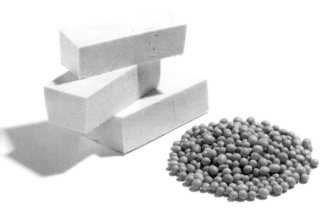

Soy comes from Asia where the Chinese have been eating this legume for centuries. Recent Western studies have shed light on the many virtues of this miraculous bean. Now, many countries around the world are rapidly integrating soy-based foods into their diets. Indeed, it has been discovered that tofu, tempeh and soy-based beverages have powerful medicinal properties, along with being rich in mineral salts, vitamins and calcium, making them ideal for arthritis sufferers. Moreover, even though research on the benefits of soy is still in the preliminary stages, the outlook is bright because their healing powers appear very promising.

Other health benefits

- Lowers cholesterol
- Promotes bowel function
- Prevents cardiovascular disease
- Lowers risk of breast and colon cancers
- Relieves menopausal symptoms
- Stabilizes blood sugar

Uses

Recent studies indicate that eating a daily serving of a soy-based food is enough to lower cancer risk.

Precautionary warning

Fermented soy products are not recommended for people sensitive to mold. Soy allergies in adult populations have intensified over recent years, probably because of the increased use of products derived from soy by the food industry. Tofu is a good source of calcium, as long as the coagulant used is calcium chloride or calcium sulfate. Read the label carefully and make sure one of those two ingredients is listed. Furthermore, some cancer experts say that women with hormone-dependent cancer, such as breast cancer, should avoid soy and its derivatives because the isoflavones and phytoestrogen they contain might promote tumor growth. This claim is particularly aimed at soy-based supplements.

Buying and storing

There are many foods made from soy: meat substitute products that mimic burgers and hot-dogs; soy flour; flavored soy beverages; tempeh; textured soy protein; and the most popular of all because it can be adapted to any recipe – tofu, available in soft and firm textures. Tofu is a bean curd made from soy milk. Once the tofu container is opened, it will keep approximately five days in the fridge, in a bowl of water that needs to be changed daily.

In the kitchen

Tofu is a veritable chameleon food, as it will take on the flavors of any foods it is prepared with. It is a good idea to marinate it before using. It is also best to not overcook it, as this will destroy its benefits. Instead, add it to the mix at the end of the cooking process. It can be used in a wide variety of dishes, from soups to desserts.

Recipes

- Banana clementine smoothie (p. 134)
  (p. 134)
- Rye flour pancakes (p. 134)
- Tortilla cups with chicken and curry (p. 179)
- Creamy cauliflower soup (p. 146)
- Pear rice pudding (p. 261)
- Cold cucumber soup (p. 149)

Good to know

From a protein point of view, soy is one of the only plant products comparable to meat, fish and eggs. The pairing of a soy food with a grain makes a complete protein – a winning combination for any vegetarian diet.

Tomato

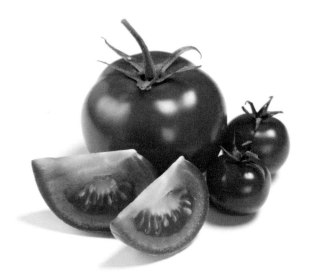

The fruit of a plant originating in Mexico, the tomato is rich in B vitamins and is full of mineral salts and trace elements. It is also an excellent source of vitamin C and provitamin A (or carotene), as well as vitamin E, an antioxidant that stimulates the body's defenses. It is low in calories and gets its vibrant red hue from lycopene, a relative of beta-carotene which has proven effective against various diseases. Contrary to popular belief, and despite its acidic taste, the tomato is alkalinizing, therefore safe for arthritis and gout sufferers.

Other health benefits

- Helps prevent appendicitis
- Lowers risk of certain cancers when cooked (colon, stomach, prostate, lung, breast and endometrial)
- Promotes digestion of starches
- Prevents cataracts

Uses

Eat daily, raw, either plain or in salads, or dried or cooked to minimize the effects of free radicals. Recent studies have proven that the tomato can lower the risk of certain types of cancer. Indeed, these reliable studies show that eating it at least seven times a week – in any form – cut the subjects' cancer risk by half. Furthermore, cooked tomato, especially in a bit of oil, contains significantly more lycopene than raw tomato. All the more reason to indulge in tomato sauce, coulis, juice, or even ketchup, to enjoy all the benefits of tomatoes.

Precautionary warning

Consumed in large amounts, the tomato can cause allergic reactions and affect the stomachs of people prone to heartburn.

Avoid eating green tomatoes, which are a frequent cause of migraines. To ripen, wrap tomatoes in newspaper and leave at room temperature for a few days. People allergic to aspirin should not eat tomatoes.

Buying and storing

Color is usually a good criterion in choosing arthritis-fighting foods. A nice, bright red, ripe tomato not only tastes better, but is also better for you with four times the carotene of a green or pale, immature tomato. They do not like to be refrigerated and will keep for a few days at room temperature.

In the kitchen

Extremely versatile, the tomato is used in many dishes, from soups to desserts, and in all manner of sauces. It is a staple in all cooking because of the delicious flavor it imparts to hot and cold dishes.

Recipes

- Black bean burrito (p. 180)
- Poached turbot with fresh tomato (p. 213)
- Fusilli with cauliflower and cherry tomatoes (p. 190)
- Macaroni and mushroom casserole with cashews (p. 190)
- Linguine with sardines (p. 212)
- Lentil moussaka (p. 201)
- Short pasta with roasted vegetables (p. 194)
- Mini lasagna rolls with pistachios and artichoke hearts (p. 197)
- Pizza with fresh tomato (p. 184)
- Tomato and chickpea soup (p. 146)
- Layered chicken and eggplant (p. 220)
- Red cabbage salad (p. 165)
- Black bean salad (p. 162)
- Pizza sauce (p. 250)
- Basic tomato sauce (p. 250)
- Winter tabbouleh with sun-dried tomato (p. 162)
- Pumpkin seed dip (p. 248)
- Sun-dried tomato dip (p. 248)

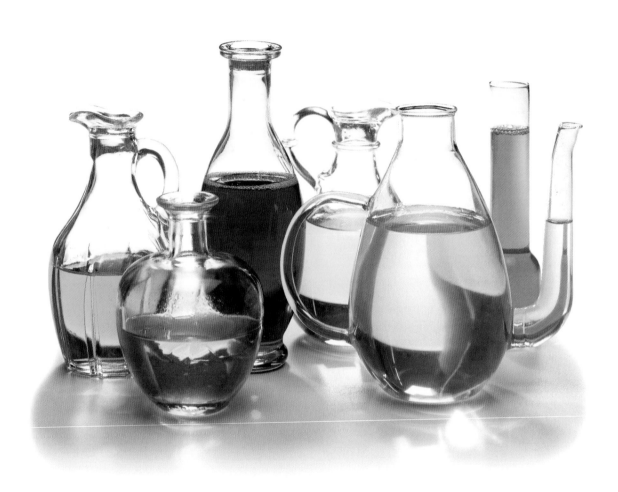

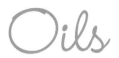

Oils

Fat is an important part of a balanced diet. Well-integrated in your diet, it allows the body to absorb fat-soluble vitamins like vitamins A, D & E. Solid fats, especially butter and lard, have a high-content of saturated fatty acids--mono and polysaturated fats. They are not recommended, as eating too much of them can be harmful to your health.

For many years, dieticians and health professionals thought they were doing a good thing by recommending we eat margarine instead of butter and lard. They had to eat crow in the early 90s and admit that they had made a mistake by not realizing that hydrogenated margarine is an important source of trans fat, a substance that raises the risk of cardiovascular disease, amongst other ill-effects. When it came to be known that many prepared foods contained these bad fats, the food industry rapidly reacted to get trans fat-free foods on the market, notably non-hydrogenated margarine which is considered safe. We have yet to know if these new offerings have any long-term effects.

Vegetable oils contain high levels of unsaturated fatty acids – mono and polyunsaturated fats in variable proportions, that are essential to good health. But vegetable oils rich in omega-6 fatty acids, such as corn, safflower and sunflower oils are not recommended for arthritis sufferers because it would seem they play a role in joint inflammation.

Many oils are rich in omega-6 but poor in omega-3, therefore, in order to prioritize the omega-3 rich oils, grapeseed, sunflower, safflower and corn oils should be replaced by olive, canola, wheat germ, flaxseed and soy oils.

To ensure an adequate daily intake of omega-3, just follow the instructions below for any of the recommended oils to accompany raw vegetables or to be used in soups. You can also get omega-3 by eating fish (see page 93). Adults' needs vary according to gender and age; children and the elderly need slightly less; and adolescents and young adults need a bit more.

Women need one of these oils daily:
½ teaspoon of flaxseed oil
2 teaspoons of canola oil
1 tablespoon of wheat germ oil
1 tablespoon of soy oil

Men need one of these oils daily:
¾ teaspoon of flaxseed oil
1 tablespoon of canola oil
4 teaspoons of wheat germ oil
4 teaspoons of soy oil

The best arthritis-fighting oils:

Canola oil

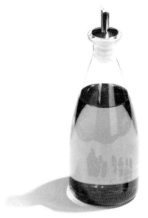

It is the oil most recommended by dieticians because of its omega-3 content, which is much superior to that of olive oil, as well as its ability to lower bad cholesterol. It is the least costly of cold-pressed oils, the most durable, and its healthy properties withstand cooking.

Arthritis benefits

Two to three teaspoons of canola oil contain more or less the required quantity of omega-3 needed each day and offer 50% of the daily requirement of vitamin E.

In the kitchen

Canola oil is used cold in vinaigrettes. Heated in a frying pan, it can be used to cook vegetables, fish and poultry. It can also be used to make cakes, breads and muffins.

Recipe

☐ Basil and pistachio pesto (p. 251)

Wheat germ oil

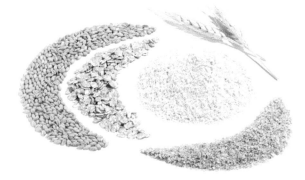

This oil is extracted from the germ by cold-pressing or with solvents. Use sparingly; it takes 15 tons of wheat to extract 4 cups of oil.

Arthritis benefits
Wheat germ oil is a good source of omega-3 and an excellent source of vitamin E.

Bonus benefit
It has anti-anemic, anti-fatigue and anti-sterility properties. It promotes growth and cellular oxygenation, protects the heart and nervous system, and is re-mineralizing.

In the kitchen
It has a robust and pleasant taste. It can be added to food, combined with olive oil or used in vinaigrettes to drizzle on roasted vegetables or salads.

Recipe
☐ Wheat germ oil vinaigrette (p. 246)

Flaxseed oil

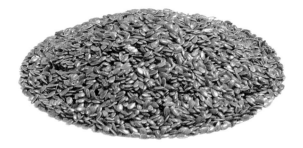

Flaxseed is particular because of its high percentage of alpha-linolenic acid – an omega-3 fatty acid.

Arthritis benefit
Because of its high omega-3 content, this oil is particularly beneficial to arthritis sufferers.

Bonus benefit
Alpha-linolenic acid is helpful in preventing cancer, improving male fertility, preventing cardiovascular disease and regulating immune function. Women taking part in a study where they had to take 2 tablespoons of flaxseed oil daily for 2 weeks stated that they suffered from fewer hot flashes and nights sweats, and less vaginal dryness. Flaxseed (see page 73) also has many virtues. Research has shown that one daily dose, as small as 2 tablespoons of ground flaxseed, can slow down tumor growth in breast cancer patients. This benefit could be due to their high lignan content, a substance known to have antiviral and anticancer properties and act as powerful antioxidants as well as regulating estrogen.

Storing
Flaxseed oil must be kept in the fridge. It will keep for four months in an unopened bottle and four weeks once the bottle has been opened.

In the kitchen

Flaxseed oil mixes very well with yogurt and with other oils for vinaigrettes. It is not appropriate for cooking, as it does not withstand heat very well. It is not recommended for use in pastry or any other oven-baked foods.

Walnut oil

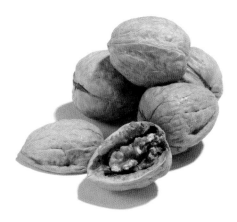

Hazelnut oil

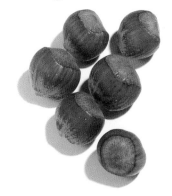

This oil is a good source of polyunsaturated fatty acids with 50% omega-6 and 12% omega-3. Its exceptional flavor is appreciated in vinaigrettes.

Arthritis benefits

With 13% alpha-linolenic acid content, it is very beneficial to arthritis sufferers.

Bonus benefit

It fortifies and promotes mental and physical capacities.

Storing

Make sure it has a best-before date on the packaging; because it is low in saturated fats, it has a very short shelf life, even in an unopened bottle.

Like olive oil, hazelnut oil is very rich in monounsaturated fatty acids, including about 8% of elaic acid. Because of this, it should be combined with an oil rich in omega-6 and omega-3. Much like walnut oil, it is appreciated by gourmets for its exquisite flavor.

Arthritis benefits

This oil is very good for arthritis sufferers because of its 11% content of omega-3 alpha-linolenic acid.

In the kitchen

Its refined taste is remarkable in vinaigrettes, it is delicious on mixed greens and raw vegetables. It can be heated at low heat in a frying pan to sauté delicate vegetables like Jerusalem artichoke and endive. It is also used in fine pastries, crepes, cookies, breads, desserts and cakes.

In the kitchen

It has a delicious flavor that makes excellent vinaigrettes. It is used to flavor cakes, and it will enhance the taste of poultry, fish and vegetables. It is not recommended for cooking.

Recipe

☐ Papaya, mango and kiwi salad infused with vanilla (p. 166)

Olive oil

Olive oil offers a high concentration (about 80%) of elaic acid, an omega-9-type unsaturated fatty acid. Omega-9 is a good fat that should be part of a balanced diet, along with omega-3 and omega-6 fatty acids. Make sure you use a first cold pressed oil that was extracted gently, without heat, to preserve its integrity.

Arthritis benefits

With an 8% alpha-linolenic acid content, olive oil is highly recommended for arthritis sufferers. Because of its prevention properties for many diseases, it is the oil I recommend the most and the one I include the most in my recipes featured in part 3.

Bonus benefit

Following a traditional Mediterranean diet (fish, fruit, vegetables) with olive oil at the forefront is beneficial for heart health. Many studies have concluded that substituting saturated fats with olive oil's monounsaturated fats, improves the ratio of good cholesterol/bad cholesterol, which in turn, prevents clogging of the blood vessels. More and more studies indicate that olive oil helps in preventing certain types of cancer, such as colon cancer. It is also used externally as a massage oil or as a beauty cream for skin and hair.

Storing

When buying first cold pressed oil, make sure you check the best-before date indicated on the label.

In the kitchen

What would Mediterranean cuisine be without olive oil? It is moderately resistant to heat, so it can also be used to grill vegetables, fish and poultry. Cold, paired with lemon juice and garlic, it will make a delicious vinaigrette, or serve it plain on raw vegetables or to dip bread in. It can be used to bake vegetable-based breads and cakes (carrot, zucchini), and is great drizzled on pizza or pasta.

Recipes

- Duck en chemise with salted herbs (p. 223)
- Quick winter pesto (p. 251)
- Potatoes with herbs and garlic (p. 238)

Sesame oil

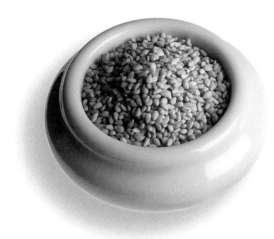

Recipes

- Asian-style artichoke (p. 169)
- Grilled salmon steak (p. 206)
- Salmon filet with ginger (p. 206)
- Cantaloupe and grape salad with ginger (p. 158)
- Mango and watercress salad (p. 170)
- Melon and avocado salad (p. 168)
- Grilled bluefin tuna in soya and ginger marinade (p. 214)

This hazelnut-tasting oil has a balanced content of 41% elaic acid and 43% omega-6 fatty acids. The sesamin and sesamolin it contains make it an excellent antioxidant.

Arthritis benefits

Sesame oil is famous for its antioxidant properties.

Bonus benefit

Asians claim that it promotes concentration and that it has detoxifying properties.

Storing

It will keep for about 18 months in a cool, dry and dark place.

In the kitchen

Its characteristic flavor will dominate in a vinaigrette and goes well with raw vegetables. Because of its overpowering taste, use it sparingly on cooked vegetables and in marinade sauces. It can be heated in a wok in small quantities for stir-fries with vegetables, poultry and fish. It the oven, it's used mostly for Asian baked goods.

Soy oil

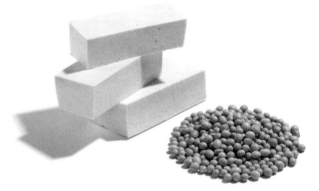

Extracted from ground soy beans, this oil retains its medicinal properties. Particularly rich in linolenic acid (omega-6) and alpha-linolenic acid (omega-3), it strengthens the immune system. It is commonly used to make margarine.

Arthritis benefits

Its concentration of alpha-linolenic acid (7%) make it a recommendable oil.

Bonus benefit

It contains lecithin, which has an anticholesteremic effect making it very good for the brain and the nervous system.

Storing

It must be kept in the fridge as soon as it is opened and used up quickly.

In the kitchen

Because it is neutral in flavor, it is used to make mixed oils, also known as vegetable oils. It is best used cold as it does not withstand heat very well.

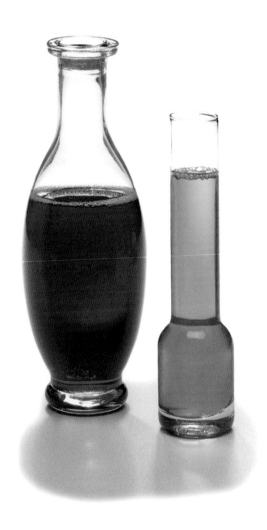

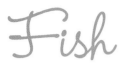

Fish

Fish is an important source of omega-3, essential fatty acids that have known anti-inflammatory properties. It is a nutritionally-sound meat substitute in a balanced diet and it is recommended to eat fish two to three times a week.

How to eat more fish

If the taste of fish does not appeal to you, try eating a more delicate-tasting fish to which you could add tomato, mushrooms, garlic and parsley. Fish cooks very quickly and makes a delicious meal or a nutritious, hearty soup. Maybe you don't eat fish because you are not familiar with this food. Try trout and salmon for a first attempt; they have a very pleasant taste, can be cooked many different ways and are sure to win you over. At first, include a fatty fish in your diet at least once a week, then work your way up to twice a week. For people with little time to spare, most fatty fish are available canned with the same health benefits. This is especially true of sardines and mackerel, a little less so for tuna, but they all make a quick meal alternative. Try them prepared in a spread to have as a pre-dinner snack with raw vegetables or crackers.

How to choose fish

The same rule applies to any fish: look for a fresh tidal smell, a bright eye, a round and shiny shape and no trace of blood around the gills or injury to the skin.

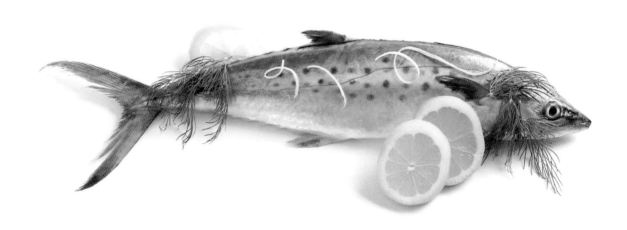

The best arthritis-fighting fish

Greenland turbot

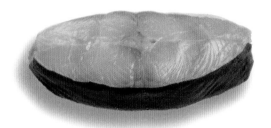

Greenland turbot is not a true turbot and actually more closely resembles its relative, halibut; however, it is sold as turbot in the United States so as not to confuse it with Pacific halibut. It is a delicate-tasting, white fish prized by gourmets..

Arthritis benefits

It is rich in omega-3 fatty acids which give it its anti-inflammatory properties.

Precautionary warning

Fish is one of the foods that causes the most allergies. People allergic to fish or seafood may have a reaction by eating a species of the same group, but not necessarily. Therefore, it is recommended that people with allergy symptoms consult an allergist before introducing new fish to their diet.

Availability

Greenland turbot is sold fresh at fish markets from March to September. It is available frozen all year long.

How to prepare

☐ Cook en papillote or poach in court bouillon.

Recipes

☐ Poached turbot with fresh tomatoes (p. 213)
☐ Quick fish soup (p. 149)

Atlantic herring

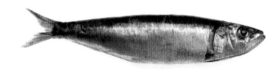

Herring are found in both the eastern and western halves of the North Atlantic Ocean. In the western Atlantic, herring range from Labrador to North Carolina. Herring is readily available cured or smoked, but is also served fresh when in season.

Arthritis benefits

Herring is rich in omega-3 fatty acids, a source of transmitter substances, such as leukotrienes and prostaglandins, that fight inflammatory reactions associated with arthritis. Herring is also rich in vitamin D which contributes to bone health and helps fight rheumatic diseases.

Precautionary warning

Cured or smoked herring is very high in salt and is not recommended for people on a low-sodium diet. 3.5 ounces of smoked or cured herring contains 900 mg of sodium, or 40% of the maximum recommended daily intake. People with gout should also avoid it, as it contains purines that provoke uric acid production.

True or false?

– Canned sardines are really herring?

True. Most canned sardines are actually small herring. "Sardine" is a generic term applied to a number of different kinds of small saltwaterfish prepared and packed in cans.

Availability

Fish markets sell fresh herring from April to September. Frozen herring is available all year long, as well as cured, marinated and smoked varieties packed in cans.

How to prepare

☐ Poached in court bouillon, oven-baked, stuffed with bread crumbs or cooked en papillote with diced tomatoes and sliced olives.

Atlantic mackerel

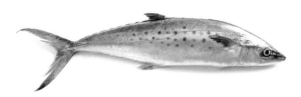

Atlantic mackerel is quite abundant, and overfishing is not occurring. It was overfished in the late 1960s and early 1970s. Authorities phased out foreign fishing and implemented annual quotas to manage U.S. fishing fleets. The stock has since rebounded to very healthy levels. Atlantic mackerel is not highly desired by most American consumers due to its rich flavor, and is more popular in foreign countries. Some of the U.S. harvest is sold fresh but most is frozen and exported to markets throughout the world.

Arthritis benefits

Along with sardines, trout, tuna, herring and salmon, Atlantic mackerel is one of the best fish sources of omega-3s, the fatty acids that promote a healthy immune system, circulation and hormonal function.

It is very nutritious and rich in selenium, a mineral useful in preventing free radicals. It is also an excellent source of vitamin D, phosphorus and magnesium which play a role in building and maintaining healthy bones.

Research

Studies have shown a link between a diet rich in fatty fish and a lower incidence of arthritis.

Omega-3 fatty acids have anti-inflammatory properties which could be useful in treating diseases like rheumatoid arthritis. It has not yet been determined how much omega-3 is required to optimize the benefits, but research indicates that 0.5 to 1.8 grams is sufficient. A 3.5 ounce serving of mackerel will yield about 1.2 grams of omega-3s.

Precautionary warning

Gout sufferers should not eat mackerel, as it is high in purines, a substance that promotes uric acid production.

True or false?
– The mercury content of fish makes it unsafe to eat.

False. Mercury's bad reputation has cast a shadow on the nutritional benefits of fish. Certain marine predators have high levels of mercury. However, mackerel's mercury levels fall well below the accepted standard of 0.5 ppm, making it safe to eat. Moreover, its levels of contaminants like polychlorobiphenyl (BPCs) are also below the accepted standard.

Availability

Fish markets sell it fresh from June to October and frozen all year long.

How to prepare

- Cook en papillote (with tomato, olives and olive oil); steamed; microwaved; grilled; stewed in broth made of green tea and lemon juice; poached in white wine, marinated and served cold.

Recipes

- Mackerel burgers (p. 178)
- Mackerel or sardine canapés (p. 166)

Sardine

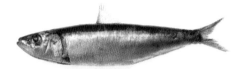

The Pacific sardine has experienced a remarkable comeback after populations dropped drastically in the 1950s. Today, this species is thriving once again. They are easy to prepare and as good for you canned as fresh.

Arthritis benefits

Sardines are a good source of inflammation-fighting omega-3 fatty acids. They also contain other nutrients such as calcium which helps in building and maintaining healthy bones.

Precautionary warning

Gout sufferers should not eat sardines as they are high in purines, a substance that promotes uric acid production.

True or false?

– Canned sardines contain more omega-3s than fresh or frozen sardines.

False. Fresh or frozen sardines have twice the omega-3 content of canned sardines.

Availability

Sardines can be found frozen in fish markets all year round.

How to prepare

☐ Use canned sardines to make canapés or sauces (see recipe). Fresh, they make a good supper served in fish broth or grilled.

Recipes

☐ Mackerel or sardine canapés (p. 166)
☐ Sardine linguine (p. 212)

Atlantic salmon

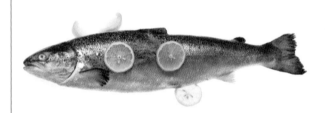

This delicious fatty fish needs no introduction, as it is abundant in our waters and on our tables, prepared in many ways and with many sauces..

Arthritis benefits

Its excellent omega-3 content give it anti-inflammatory properties. It is rich in vitamin D for good bone health. It is one of the fattiest of fatty fish but it still contains less fat than red meat and its fat is healthy.

Precautionary warning

Salmon is often served raw or marinated. Raw, smoked or marinated fish can contain bacteria, viruses or parasites that can only be killed with cooking. People most sensitive to food poisoning – young children , immunosuppressed persons or pregnant women – should avoid these types of salmon.

True or false?

– Eating farmed salmon can be harmful to your health..

False. Results of a 2004 Science magazine international study pointed the finger at farmed salmon as being potentially harmful. Another study in 2005 came to the same conclusion, revealing that farmed salmon contained high levels of organochlorine contaminants such as DDT and BCPs. But, according to some researchers, these findings are unnecessarily alarmist. Furthermore, researchers from the Harvard School of Public Health state that the benefits of eating fish far outweigh the risks.

Availability

Farmed salmon is available all year round, fresh or frozen, in supermarkets. Wild salmon is readily available at fish markets.

Storing

Eat on the same day it's purchased or freeze for no longer than one month.

How to prepare

☐ Raw, in gravlax or tartare. Cooked en papillote with lemon and tarragon. In the microwave in a teriyaki-style marinade. Oven-grilled or on an electric barbecue. Poached whole in white wine, then served cold with a yogurt sauce. Canned salmon can be used on pizza, in sandwiches and salads, or with pasta.

Recipes

☐ Stuffed avocados infused with lemon and curry (canned) (p. 160)
☐ Squash stuffed with salmon and rice (canned) (p. 176)
☐ Grilled salmon steaks (p. 206)
☐ Ginger salmon fillets (p. 206)
☐ Salmon fillets en chemise (p. 208)
☐ Salmon pasta salad (canned) (p. 180)
☐ Salmon imperial triangles (canned) (p. 161)

Tuna

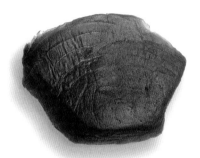

Do not confuse canned albacore tuna with bluefin tuna, a fatty fish available fresh from July to September, to the delight of all gourmets. Bluefin tuna is prized for its excellent meat, rich in omega-3 fatty acids, making it very beneficial for arthritis sufferers.

Arthritis benefits

Tuna is rich in selenium, an important mineral supporting antioxidant enzymes in the fight against free radicals. It is an excellent source of vitamins A & D, both contributing to bone health. A 3.5 ounce serving of bluefin tuna, canned albacore or yellowtail tuna will yield respectively, 1.4, 0.9 or 0.3 grams of omega-3s.

True or false?
– Grilled fish is healthier than fried fish.

True. Studies have revealed that subjects 65 years and older who ate one or two servings of grilled fish a week had a lower incidence of cardiovascular disease than those subjects who ate the same amount of fried fish.

Availability
Sold fresh at fish markets from July to September.

How to prepare
Fresh:
- Cooked in the oven à la niçoise with tomato and olives. Skewered on an electric barbecue. In a ceviche with lime juice. Grilled (see recipe).

Canned:
- In sandwiches, with tomato and olives. In fish soup. In salads, with capers and anchovies.

Tip
If cooked too long, tuna will dry out: it is ready to serve as soon as the meat turns opaque.

Recipe
- Grilled bluefin tuna, marinated in soy and ginger (p. 214)

Lake trout or rainbow trout

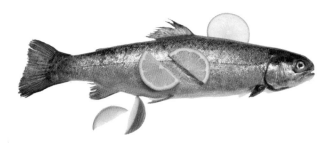

Fisherman love the delicate taste and texture of lake trout. Rainbow trout, though not as refined-tasting, is also very popular.

Arthritis benefits
Trout is a fatty or semi-fatty fish that usually contains a fair amount of omega-3 fatty acids. It also contains phosphorus, which helps promote bone health, and selenium, which helps fight free radicals.

Precautionary warning
Lake trout contains high levels of mercury but as long as it is only consumed occasionally, it poses little risk. People who eat it often should cut back and only eat two 8 ounce servings a month. This restriction does not apply to other kinds of trout.

True or false?
– Wild trout is healthier than farmed trout..

True. Researchers have found that wild trout is richer in omega-3s than farmed trout because of its diet.

Availability

At the supermarket or fish market, fresh or frozen.

How to prepare

☐ Cooked en papillote, with fresh herbs and almonds. Grilled in the oven or on the barbecue.

Recipes

☐ Trout fillets with green peppercorns and curry sauce (p. 210)
☐ Trout fillets with almond tartar sauce (p. 209)

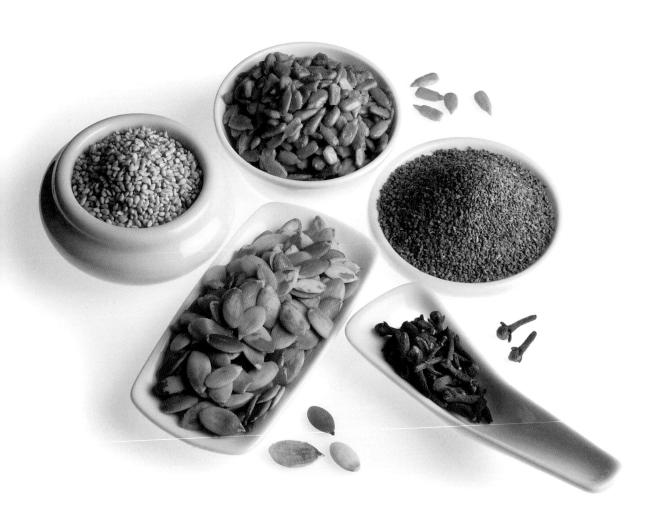

Herbs and spices

Herbs and spices take center stage in my kitchen. If, like me, you love aromatics, do not hesitate to mix up your own personal spice blend (see page 252) to have on hand whenever you fancy cooking flavorful food.

We owe a lot to herbs and spices: they are at the heart of all cooking, they give essence and aroma to cooked foods, turning plain ingredients into veritable feasts. Imagine spaghetti sauce with no bay leaf or oregano; tabbouleh devoid of parsley; guacamole sans jalapeno; Thai stir-fry missing chili pepper; pesto longing for basil; you might as well make curry without...well, curry.

What we know the least about these aromatics are their surprising properties. Most herbs and spices are rich in vitamins, but many also have antioxidant and anti-inflammatory properties able to diminish and soothe joint pain.

Take celery seeds for example: not only do they contain polyacetylenes, substances potentially beneficial in the fight against cancer, they also contain apigenin, a substance that efficiently fights free radicals by acting as rust-proofing for the joints. Sage, for its part, contains vitamin K, which contributes to bone health and has important anti-inflammatory properties. Furthermore, studies have shown that sage may help in slowing down the aging process by improving neurotransmission in the brain. Chili pepper, one of many spices with amazing medicinal properties, contains analgesic substances that can diminish pain signals to the brain.

Herbs and spices share their health-boosting properties through flavoring the dishes they're used in. Oregano, tarragon, rosemary and cumin are excellent alternatives to salt for people restricted by a low-sodium diet, or who do not tolerate such foods as garlic and onion.

The best cancer fighting herbs and spices

Clove

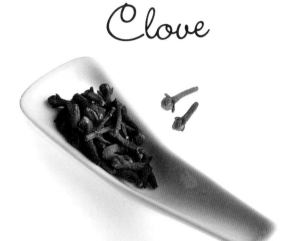

This strong and acrid spice is native to the Moluccas islands in Indonesia, also known as Spice Islands. It is the dried flower bud of a tree from the myrtle family and looks like a small tack. Clove shares the same arthritis-fighting properties as ginger. Its medicinal virtues are age-old, with a proven track record fighting viruses, infections and pain. Even to this day, it is used in preparing many medications throughout the world.

Other health benefits
- Helps eliminate intestinal parasites
- Boosts immune system
- Helps heal sores, in lotion form
- Prevents congestion and aids breathing
- Promotes white blood cell production
- Prevents infectious diseases

Precautionary warning
Clove essential oil can be very dangerous if ingested; never replace cloves with clove essential oil.

In the kitchen

Its slightly spicy taste flavors stews and jams. It goes particularly well with apple.

Home remedies

A compress of clove water can offer soothing relief for burns or mild pain. Rinsing your mouth with clove water can soothe a tooth ache. You can also rub a whole clove into the gums to relieve such pain as teething pain in babies.

Recipes

- Quick oatmeal cookies (p. 264)
- Duck en chemise with salted herbs (p. 223)
- Tea-and ginger-flavored kiwi compote (p. 130)
- Quick tea jam (p. 132)
- Duck thigh with dried fruit (p. 224)
- Lentil and fruit picadillo with golden pita (p. 193)
- Buckwheat and mushroom terrine (p. 164)

Good to know

The smell of cloves repels moths and mosquitoes. Stud an orange with whole cloves to make a natural deodorizer for your closet.

Turmeric

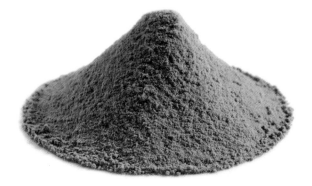

Used for centuries in Ayurvedic medicine, turmeric is rich in vitamin C, iron and potassium. It is also known as Indian saffron because of its yellow hue which it gets from curcumin, its active ingredient. But its resemblance with saffron stops there, having a flavor that's both slightly bitter and quite a bit spicier. Turmeric has antioxidant and anti-inflammatory properties making it highly recommended for arthritis sufferers.

Other health benefits

- Antiseptic
- Antispasmodic
- Lowers risk of cancer, especially skin cancer
- Facilitates digestion
- Prevents cataracts
- Prevents Alzheimer's disease
- Heals skin conditions
- Relieves diarrhea
- Anti-parasitic

Home remedy

Using ½ teaspoon three times a week in soups, vegetable dishes, and stews will help relieve joint pain.

Precautionary warning

Caution is recommended in cases of gastric ulcers, as one study shows that high doses of curcumanoids may irritate the stomach.

Buying and storing

It is best to buy in small quantities as turmeric's beneficial properties wear out quite fast.

In the kitchen

This spice, which is also used as a dye in India, gives flavor and color to curries (in garam masala), soups, rice and meat stews. .

Recipes

- Stuffed avocados infused with lemon and curry (p. 160)
- Orange-flavored beets (p. 234)
- Mackerel or sardine canapés (p. 166)
- Chickpea and vegetable curry (p. 200)
- Tortilla cups with chicken and curry (p. 179)
- Carrot ginger soup (p. 142)
- Green pea soup (p. 144)
- Creamy cauliflower soup (p. 146)
- Celery soup with turmeric (p. 150)
- Parsnip, carrot and sweet potato soup (p. 240)
- Sweet potato and apple mash (p. 240)
- Apple-and orange-infused rice (p. 241)
- Carrot and beet salad (p. 165)
- Cabbage and apple salad (p. 183)
- Curried fruit salad (p. 265)
- Endive and fennel salad with apple (p. 169)
- Clementine and turmeric sauce (p. 130)
- Orange curry vinaigrette (p. 246)

Good to know

Darker colored turmeric is a sign of quality.

Ginger

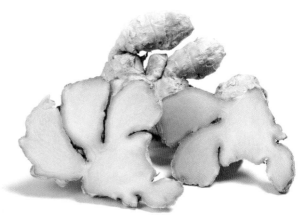

For centuries, Asian people have been cooking with this rhizome, known for its infection-fighting properties. It is widely used in Europe to fight nausea, more particularly in Germany, where it was first used against motion sickness. It is also efficient in relieving joint pain, headaches and colds. Even though its flavor is characteristic of Asian cuisine, it is more and more present in Western cooking.

Other health benefits

- Anticoagulant
- Antiseptic
- Prevents flatulence
- Prevents ulcers
- Stimulates digestion

Cold-fighting home remedy

At the first signs of flu or cold, boil two slices of fresh ginger in one cup of water and let steep for 10 minutes; add a sprinkling of cinnamon. This tea will also help relieve joint pain, stomach ailments and promote digestion..

Precautionary warning

Consumed in large quantities, ginger may cause diarrhea. As with many things, moderation is the best policy. If ginger is not already a part of your diet, introduce it gradually. It will help fight morning sickness in pregnant women, but it should be limited to 2 grams per day.

Buying and storing
Look for long, firm rhizomes with clear, silvery skin; size is a sign of maturity, indicating good fibre content. Keep ginger at room temperature. It also freezes well, whole or grated.

In the kitchen
Ginger's delicate but tingly taste is very versatile: from soups to entrées, stews, curries, sauces, vinaigrettes, vegetables dishes all the way to desserts and hot beverages. It comes in all shapes and manners: fresh, powdered, candied, dried, in syrup, ground or in marmalade, but its therapeutic properties are at their best when fresh. Grating it is a good way to release all of its healthy substances.

Good combination
Its flavor pairs itself really well with cilantro, lemon and orange. Add thin strips to a vegetable salad for a tasty boost of vitamins and fiber with very few calories.

Recipes
- Asian style artichokes (p. 169)
- Chickpea and vegetable curry (p. 200)
- Duck thigh with dried fruit (p. 224)
- Tea-and ginger-flavored kiwi compote (p. 130)
- Quick tea jam (p. 132)
- Gingered salmon filets (p. 206)
- Orange and ginger rabbit (p. 228)
- Orange and ginger muffins (p. 132)
- Carrot and ginger soup (p. 142)
- Cantaloupe and grape salad with ginger (p. 158)
- Cabbage and apple salad (p. 183)
- Curried fruit salad (p. 265)
- Clementine and turmeric sauce (p. 130)
- Orange and curry vinaigrette (p. 246)

Good to know
Commercial ginger ale contains very little actual ginger and does not offer much in terms of medicinal properties. However, it is very easy to make your own ginger beer: boil ¾ cup of peeled ginger pieces in 4 cups of water for 30 minutes. Sweeten with 1 or 2 tablespoons of honey, to taste. A dose of 1 or 2 grams of ginger powder is equivalent to about 10 grams of fresh ginger, or to a ¼-inch slice of a medium-sized rhizome..

Celery seeds

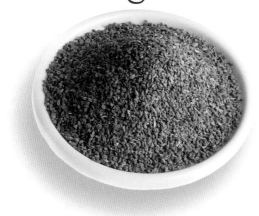

Traces of these aromatic seeds have been found in ancient Egyptian tombs. They give a slightly bitter, unique flavor to many dishes. They contain polyacetylenes, potentially beneficial cancer-fighting substances, as well as apigenin, a powerful antioxidant which battles free radicals. It was once thought to fight edema and jaundice. Today, it is consumed in small doses to fight gout and rheumatism.

Other health benefits
- Fights urinary tract inflammation
- Lowers blood pressure
- Stimulates digestion

Uses
To make celery seed tea, put 2.5 ml of ground seeds in one cup of hot water.

In the kitchen
They give lovely flavor to broths, soups, stews and boiled dinners; they give extra flavor to curries and garam masala. Their flavor is enhanced by dry-roasting them before grinding.

Recipes
- Creamy cauliflower soup (p. 146)
- Spiced rice with sweet peppers (p. 241)

Parsley

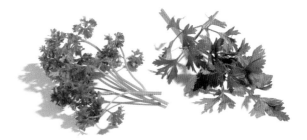

This aromatic plant is often used as a mere garnish, but it is a very healthful food with many medicinal benefits, including maintaining joint health and mobility. Parsley is rich in vitamins A, B, C and calcium, making it very good for arthritis sufferers.

Other health benefits
- Antiseptic
- Diuretic
- Prevents flatulence
- Protects against certain types of cancer
- Freshens your breath
- Relieves menstrual discomfort
- Tonic
- Anti-parasitic

Uses
Raw parsley should be eaten daily in salads or hors-d'oeuvres because of its medicinal properties and nutritional value.

Precautionary warning
Overeating parsley could be harmful to pregnant women as it contains substances that stimulate contractions.

Buying and storing
Most supermarkets offer both curly-leaf and flat-leaf parsley. It keeps well in the fridge as long as it is fresh and kept dry. Remove the leaves that wilt and turn yellow.

In the kitchen

You can chop the stems and leaves to flavor vinaigrettes and add crispness to salads and cold dishes. It can also be added to flavor stews, pasta and rice.

Recipes

- Squash stuffed with salmon and rice (p. 176)
- Salmon filets en chemise (p. 208)
- Trout filets with green peppercorns and curry sauce (p. 210)
- Poached turbot with fresh tomato (p. 213)
- Cauliflower and cherry tomato fusilli (p. 190)
- Macaroni casserole with mushrooms and cashews (p. 190)
- Linguine with sardines (p. 212)
- Meatless shepherd's pie (p. 192)
- Pasta with sweet pepper coulis (p. 196)
- Basil and pistachio pesto (p. 251)
- Winter pesto (p. 251)
- Layered chicken and eggplant (p. 220)
- Parsnip, carrot and sweet potato mash (p. 240)
- Clementine and carrot salad with sage (p. 160)
- Salmon pasta salad (p. 180)
- Winter vegetable soup (p. 153)
- Quick minestrone (p. 148)
- Winter tabbouleh with sundried tomatoes (p. 162)
- Pumpkin seed dip (p. 248)
- Salmon imperial triangles (p. 161)

Good to know

25 grams of fresh parsley will yield 50 mg of vitamin C, representing nearly 80% of the daily recommended intake.

Chili peppers

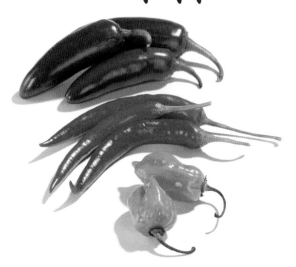

All peppers are not created equal – don't confuse the sweet ones with the hot ones (even though one taste will quickly clear things up!). The chili pepper owes its heat to a substance that affects mucus membranes much like a decongestant. It contains more vitamin C than an orange but it does not have much of an impact on the daily recommended intake because of the limited quantity most people can consume at a time. It also contains an analgesic substance that interrupts neural transmission of pain signals in the brain. Capsaicin is responsible for most of the pepper's properties, and is the substance that gives it heat and its decongestant and expectorant powers. Moreover, the heat caused by capsaicin forces the body to produce endorphins, triggering a calming sensation which might explain chili pepper's addictive appeal.

Other health benefits

- Improves blood flow
- Clears airways
- Lowers blood pressure
- Lowers risk of cardiovascular disease
- Reduces chronic bronchitis symptoms

- Stimulates digestion
- May prevent certain types of cancer
- Prevents coagulation
- Lowers cholesterol
- Stimulates endorphin secretion

Precautionary warning

You should never apply pepper-based essential oils to your skin. Chili peppers raise gastric acidity and irritate the digestive tract, especially near the anus. To benefit from their properties, it is recommended to add them to your diet gradually. Experts are still at odds about the effect of chili pepper on stomach ulcers; some say they aggravate them and intensify the pain, others say the opposite. It is best to judge for yourself. Because they irritate eyes and skin, it is recommended to wear gloves when manipulating chili peppers, or at least wash your hands with warm, soapy water often after touching them.

Buying and storing

Fresh chili peppers keep well in the fridge. They provide benefits whether dried or crushed, but even in these formats, they should be kept in the fridge or the freezer to preserve their properties.

In the kitchen

The hottest ones are the habanero and the japones; the mildest are the anaheim and the paprika peppers.

The dark green finger-sized jalapeno's taste changes from one pepper to another. Add any of these peppers to flavor broths, soups, vinaigrettes, marinades, sauces or stews to your taste and heat tolerance.

Recipes

- Asian style artichoke (p. 169)
- Chickpea and vegetable curry (p. 200)
- Grapefruit, avocado and fennel cup (p. 170)
- Tortilla cup with chicken and curry (p. 179)
- Cauliflower and cherry tomato fusilli (p. 190)
- Lentil moussaka (p. 201)
- Pasta with sweet pepper coulis (p. 196)
- Short pasta with roasted vegetables (p. 194)
- Lentil and fruit picadillo with golden pita (p. 193)
- Tomato and chickpea soup (p. 146)
- Celery soup with turmeric (p. 150)
- Quinoa with cherries and nuts (p. 238)
- Spicy rice with sweet peppers (p. 241)
- Mango and watercress salad (p. 170)
- Papaya, mango and kiwi salad infused with vanilla (p. 166)
- Pumpkin seed dip (p. 248)
- Sundried tomato dip (p. 248)

Good to know

Dried chili peppers are usually hotter than fresh ones. Smaller peppers contain more seeds and membranes, making them hotter.

Sage

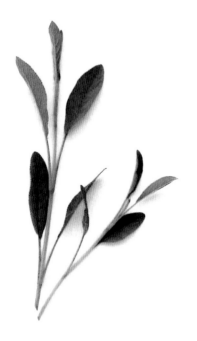

Sage has a long history of medicinal and culinary use and has been grown for centuries for its food and healing properties. It used to be said that if you had sage in the garden, you didn't need a doctor. It is one of the richest herbs in antioxidants. It contains vitamin K which helps build and maintain healthy bones and has anti-inflammatory properties. Studies have shown that it may play a role in slowing the aging process by improving neural transmission in the brain.

Other health benefits

- Improves and stimulates digestion
- Relieves hot flashes and other menopausal symptoms
- Fights depression
- Relieves nerve fatigue
- Regulates sweating
- Treats throat infection

Home remedies

Throat-wash to relieve a sore throat
Pour 2 teaspoons of dried sage and ½ teaspoon of salt into 8.5 ounces of boiling water. Remove from heat, cover and let steep 10 minutes. Filter and gargle while tepid. Repeat throughout the day.

Sage tea
It is best used dried when its flavor is strongest. Put 20 grams of dried sage leaves into 4 cups of water, boil 5 minutes. Steep for 5 minutes and filter. Drink a small glass before meals. Used externally, sage tea is antiseptic, a cicatrizant and a decongestant. You can also use it in a compress applied to sores, ulcers, contusions and inflammation.

In the kitchen
Use it fresh to enhance salads, vegetables dishes and pasta, and give flavor to oils and vinegars.

Recipes
- Orange and ginger rabbit (p. 228)
- Squash and fennel soup (p. 152)
- Clementine and carrot salad with sage (p. 160)
- Winter vegetable soup (p. 153)
- Quick minestrone (p. 148)

Seeds

The miracle of life occurs every time a seed germinates. All it requires are air and water to develop all that hides within, into a condensed package of health-providing vitamins, minerals and other nutrients – all in a matter of days. Depending on the variety, a few spoonfuls of sprouted seeds will give a good quantity of vegetable protein, vitamins A & B and lots of vitamin C.

Sprouted seeds can be eaten raw in salads, sandwiches and spring rolls, or they can be added to soups and stews. All manner of seeds, grains, beans and legumes can be sprouted:

- Grain: wheat, kamut, farro, buckwheat, millet, rye, barley
- Beans and legumes: kidney bean, chickpea, lentil, soy
- Vegetable: cabbage, leek, arugula, and more.

What to do

All you need is a glass jar, a square of muslin or cheesecloth, an elastic and some water. Seeds like alfalfa and soy beans need more space, so just use a few. But seeds like chickpea, lentil, wheat and farro need little space so you can use more.

Place a small quantity of seeds in a glass jar that will hold 4 cups of water. Cover them with spring water and let soak overnight.

The next day, cover the jar's opening with the cloth, held in place with the elastic.

Run tap water over the covered opening, rinsing the seeds until the water is no longer green, then drain. To drain well, shake the seeds so they will adhere to the wall of the jar that you will sit on its side. Repeat the rinsing process 2 to 3 times a day. Keep out of the light.

After a few days, from 1 to 6 depending on the seeds, sprouts should be visible. Then place the jar in a sunlit place to encourage the seeds to produce chlorophyll, a source of vitamin A.

Make sure you rinse the seeds at least twice a day until sprouting occurs.

When the sprouts have emerged, the seeds are ready to eat. Keep in the fridge uncovered no longer than one day.

The fastest-sprouting seeds – often overnight – are squash, sesame, sunflower, almond, hazelnut, quinoa and fenugreek. They only require 5 to 14 hours of soaking. The sprout is barely visible, the seeds tender and light-tasting, except in the case of sesame and fenugreek. Sunflower seeds will keep for 2 days; sesame, quinoa and almond will keep a little longer, as long as no stagnant water is left standing in the jar.

The best arthritis-fighting seeds

Pumpkin

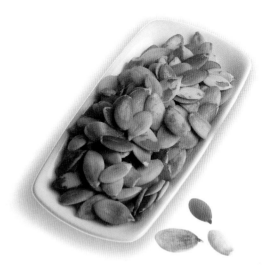

The seeds of this winter squash (see page 68) are rich in amino-acids: alanine, glycine and glutamic acid. They contain magnesium, linoleic acid (omega-6), copper and phosphorus, but it is their high zinc concentration that makes them favorable for arthritis sufferers, as zinc helps promote immune reaction.

Other health benefits
- Lowers risk of kidney stones
- Laxative
- Relieves bladder irritation and urination problems related to benign enlarged prostate
- Anti-parasitic

Recipe
- Pumpkin seed dip (p. 248)

Sprouting
(For ¼ cup of seeds)
Soaking time: 12 hours
Sprouting time: 24 hours
Sprout height at harvest: minuscule

Sesame

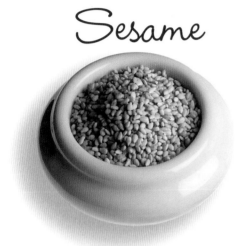

The sesame seed's zinc content makes it valuable, as zinc plays a role in a strong immune system by helping t-lymphocyte production. Researchers have discovered that a slight zinc deficiency seems to diminish immune protection and cause various infections. Combined with vitamin C, zinc is even more efficient in preventing colds and infections.

Buying and storing
Some health food stores sell unhulled black and beige sesame seeds; grocery stores mainly sell white hulled seeds. From a nutritional point of view, the unhulled variety is much better than the hulled. Kept in a dry, cool and dark place, they will last at least one year. Sesame seed paste, or tahini, is easy to find in most supermarkets, health food stores and Asian markets.

In the kitchen
Heating the seeds will enhance their flavor. Simply toast in a dry frying pan or spread on a baking sheet and put in the oven for a few minutes at 220°F. They are delicious in a salad, stir-fry, soup or pâté. They offer even more nutrients when sprouted. Theses should be eaten as soon as they're sprouted because they quickly develop a bitter taste.

Recipes
- Beets infused with orange (p. 234)
- Grapefruit, avocado and fennel cup (p. 170)
- Grilled salmon steaks (p. 206)
- Honey and almond flakes (p. 137)
- Pizza with goat cheese and pesto (p. 178)
- Clementine and carrot salad with sage (p. 160)
- Mango and watercress salad (p. 170)
- Salmon pasta salad (p. 180)

Sprouting
(For ¼ cup of unhulled seeds)
Soaking time: 4-6 hours
Sprouting time: 24-36 hours
Sprout height at harvest: minuscule

Sunflower

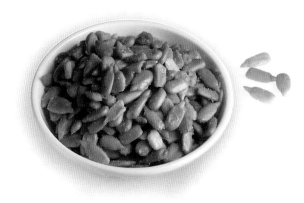

The sunflower is a plant native to the Americas, cultivated by indigenous Americans for hundreds of years, even before they discovered squash, beans and corn. Its seeds contain a cornucopia of vitamins, but no vitamin C. Its high S-Adenosyl-methionine (SAMe) content is what gives it remarkable anti-pain and anti-inflammatory properties.

Precautionary warning

If you have trouble digesting sunflower seeds, soak then overnight before eating, this will make then more alkaline and digestible.

Buying and storing

Unshelled, they will keep for months in the pantry or the fridge. Shelled, they are best kept in the fridge or the freezer.

Tip

They are easy to shell if you put them in a Ziplock-type plastic bag and crush them lightly with a rolling pin before immersing them in a bowl of water; the seeds will sink down to the bottom and all you have to do then is scoop out the shells, drain and dry the seeds on a paper towel.

In the kitchen

They are good to snack on, like nuts, or add them to cereal, fruit or vegetable salads, or cakes. You can use them instead of pine nuts to make pesto; add them to your stuffing and stews; or use them to make breading.

Recipes

- Quick oatmeal cookies (p. 264)
- Nut burgers (p. 182)
- Honey and almond flakes (p. 137)

Sprouting

(For ½ cup of unhulled seeds)
Soaking time: 4-8 hours
Sprouting time: 1-2 days
Sprout height at harvest: up to 12 mm

Good to know

Native Americans used sunflower seeds to make dye in fabric- and basket-making. They used the stem of the plant as a building material.

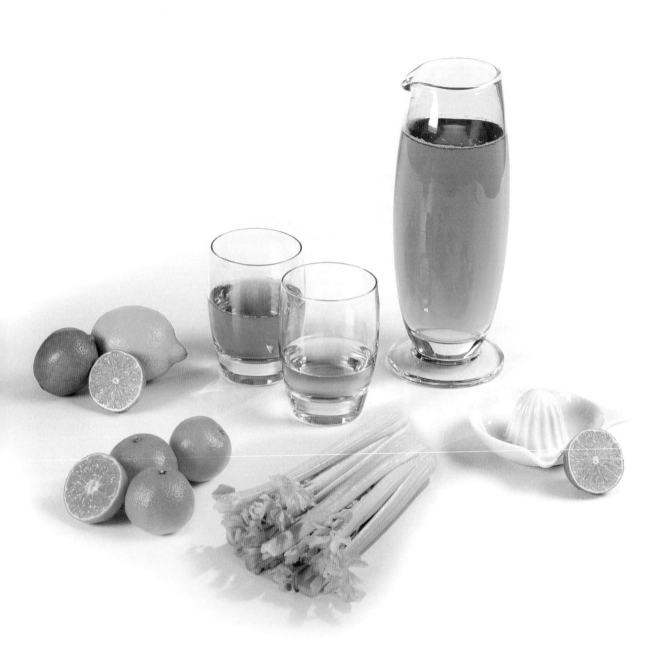

Beverages

Most fruits and vegetables, and even some grains, can be used to extract juice that is very healthy and beneficial. Fresh juice is often easier to digest than the food it came from and is of much better quality than anything available commercially, where the ingredients have been treated, transformed, pasteurized and added to until there is very little left of the original version. With a good juicer, fresh juice will contain maximum nutrients to sustain and improve health.

Fresh juice has long been known for its therapeutic properties:

- Celery juice promotes good digestion and relieves arthritis pain;
- Carrot juice treats stomach discomfort and hyperacidity;
- Valerian juice aids sleep and reduces stress;
- St. John's wort juice fights depression, overti-redness, neuralgia, headaches and rheumatism.

Vegetable juice is made using the entire vegetable: leaves, stem, roots (except for rhubarb and carrots leaves, which are toxic raw), in order to get the most nutrients.

Different taste combinations will delight you. Try adding carrot or celery to other vegetable juices, or mixing different varieties of the same vegetable. The combinations below are most beneficial to arthritis sufferers and constitute many of the same combinations I suggest in the recipe section for soups and salads:

- Carrot, cucumber, celery
- Garlic, carrot, celery, watercress, shallot, parsley, red sweet pepper, tomato (a home-made garden cocktail)
- Beet, carrot, sweet pepper, apple
- Beet, carrot, cucumber
- Spinach, celery, parsley, carrot
- Cabbage, apple, lemon
- Grapefruit, orange, honey
- Cantaloupe, cherry (strawberry or blueberry)

Fresh blender vegetable juice for one

In blender, add 1 slice of red onion; 1 carrot, brushed clean and cut in pieces; a few celery leaves; 2 or 3 spinach leaves, washed; 2 or 3 arugula leaves, washed; and 3 cherry tomatoes, halved. Blend for 5 seconds, add ½ cup of cold water (or any liquid, like vegetable juice or vegetable cooking water) and pulse for another 5 seconds. Salt and pepper to taste, and strain.

Tea

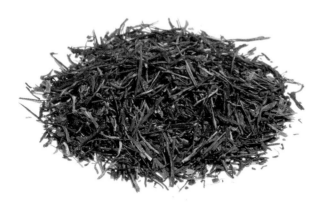

Tea is the most popular drink in the world. More than 4,000 years ago, the Chinese already knew of tea's therapeutic properties and believed it to relieve joint pain. It also promotes good digestion and a recent study suggests that tea inhibits certain types of cancers, and protects against cardiovascular disease. Tea is low in calories, providing you don't add sugar or milk, and low in sodium.

Other health benefits

- Lowers blood pressure
- Temporarily improves cognitive function
- Fights atherosclerosis
- Lowers cancer risk
- Cures diarrhea
- Promotes good digestion
- Kills viruses and bacteria
- Prevents tooth decay and periodontitis

Uses

A cup of tea at break-time is better for you than a cup of coffee for its therapeutic properties. But tea also contains caffeine (theine) so it is best to limit consumption to three cups a day.

Precautionary warning

Tannins in tea may inhibit absorption of certain food minerals, such as iron. To counteract this, drink tea in between meals with a bit of lemon juice, or add more iron-rich foods to your diet.

Drinking a lot of tea may stain the teeth. Because of the effects of theine, it is recommended that pregnant women abstain from drinking tea. Nursing women should drink it in moderation, as it might interfere with baby's sleep. It is not recommended to let babies and children drink tea, because they might react badly to tannins and theine.

Buying and storing

Amongst the most popular teas are black tea (darjeeling, breakfast tea), oolong (made from partially dried and heated green leaves), and green tea with its more bitter, but just as refreshing, taste. Tea keeps well in a dark, airtight container but never keep it in the fridge, as the cold will kill its aromas.

In the kitchen

The ideal digestive beverage, tea is a perfect way to end a meal.

Recipes

- Kiwi, tea and ginger compote (p. 130)
- Quick green tea jam (p. 132)
- Duck thighs with dried fruit (p. 224)

Good to know

Tea in bags contains just as much antioxidant power as loose tea. To benefit from all of tea's virtues, make sure you steep it for approximately 3 minutes, whether in bags or loose.

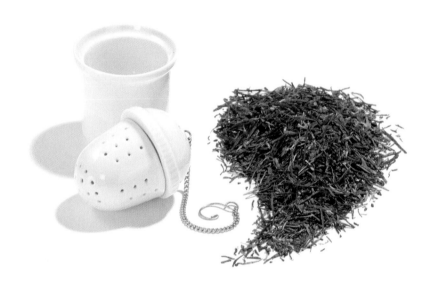

Part Three

Cooking for pleasure

Eating and cooking are two of life's greatest pleasures. For me, they go together like milk and cookies–or should I say like tomatoes and cucumbers! They are not separate activites; one rarely happens without the other. That does not mean I don't enjoy going out to eat, either at a restaurant or at a friend's house. Quite the opposite, I find it very inspiring to eat someone else's cooking and be in another kitchen. These out-of-kitchen experiences feed my imagination, my thirst for new ideas, my taste for discovering new foods and flavors. You can't get all that by sticking to your own territory; you must go and take a peek–and a sniff–in other pots and pans.

Cooking, besides the pleasure of preparing food and the satisfaction of seeing the result, fulfills a need that we all share: to be creative and to try new things. In this spirit, I hope the recipes I've created will serve as a launch pad for your own creativity. While I've put in a lot of effort to make healthy and tasty recipes that will please the most discerning palates, I hope this work is not in vain and is appreciated. Nevertheless, taste is a very personal sense, intertwined with identity, family and background. Use all of these to modify recipes and add ingredients; the end results will have your signature on it. Use the knowledge and information gathered in the first part of this book to guide you as you look for the foods that will relieve your pain, make you healthier, and give you pleasure.

Recipe ingredients

In the case of an ingredient that does not work for you, a substitution will be in order.
For example, if you are allergic to **soy milk** (I use it often), and usually use **cow's milk**, feel free to replace one for the other. The same goes for **whole wheat pastry flour**; it is the one I prefer but it might not suit you. It was only natural for me to pick and choose foods that we, as a couple, thought worked best for us. In soups, I tend to go overboard with **zucchini** because I really like it; you can replace it with a lesser quantity of **potato**. **Tamari sauce** can replace **soy sauce, chives** or **basil** can replace **cilantro**, and so on. The foods will still be tasty, you will feel better, and you will put your own spin on the meal you serve to your family. Whether or not you are following a recipe, cooking is always better with a bit of imagination and a dash of boldness.

In order to create the recipes in part 3, I gathered all the foods that were known to have real benefits for the treatment of joint pain, and I avoided those that were iffy or problematic. You will notice very little meat and an abundance of fruits and vegetables. Eating should always be pleasurable, so I occasionaly strayed from the Swiss model against arthritis (see page 24), to propose some poultry recipes that could come in handy when entertaining. As with my previous book, I follow one rule throughout all my recipes, the EHT rule: Easy, Healthy, Tasty. Keeping in mind that a lot of people have little time to spend in the kitchen, I use fresh fruits and vegetables and foods that you are likely to have on hand most anytime. To help, here is a list of foods often used in my recipes so you can keep your pantry and fridge well stocked.

The arthritis sufferer's grocery list

In the pantry
- [ ] Canned fish: sockeye salmon, sardines in olive oil, mackerel, tuna
- [ ] Canned legumes: chickpeas, white, red and black kidney beans, lentils
- [ ] Canned vegetables: tomatoes, tomato paste, beets, roasted sweet pepper, cream corn, kernel corn
- [ ] Garlic, shallot, onion
- [ ] Fresh ginger
- [ ] Dried tomato
- [ ] Canned chicken broth
- [ ] Dried fruit: apricots, strawberries, cranberries, figs, golden raisins
- [ ] Spices: cinnamon, clove, turmeric, coriander, cumin, hot pepper flakes, fennel seeds, cajun spices, paprika, chili mix, nutmeg
- [ ] Dried herbs: thyme, mint, basil, oregano, tarragon, sage
- [ ] Rice: long-grain white or brown, basmati
- [ ] Quinoa, millet, white buckwheat (available in health food stores)
- [ ] Regular rolled oats, texturized soy protein
- [ ] Organic whole wheat pastry flour (finer than regular flour), cornmeal, buckwheat flour, baking powder
- [ ] Pasta: spaghetti, short pasta, soup pasta
- [ ] Cold-pressed extra-virgin olive oil, canola oil
- [ ] Tamari sauce, Dijon mustard, cider vinegar, balsamic vinegar
- [ ] Unsweetened regular or vanilla flavored soy milk, or rice milk
- [ ] Natural peanut butter
- [ ] Honey, raw sugar, brown sugar

In the fridge
- [ ] Citrus: clementines, oranges, lemons and limes
- [ ] Cheese: parmesan, gruyere, low-fat cheese
- [ ] Walnut oil or hazelnut oil, sesame oil
- [ ] Basic vegetables: carrots, cabbage, rutabaga
- [ ] Non-hydrogenated margarine

- [ ] Eggs
- [ ] Black olives packed in oil
- [ ] Various lettuces and herbs (parsley, chives)
- [ ] Flour tortillas
- [ ] Plain yogurt

In the freezer
- [ ] Various nuts: almonds, hazelnuts, pecans, pine nuts, pistachios
- [ ] Various seeds: pumpkin, flax, sunflower, sesame
- [ ] Vegetable broth (p. 144)
- [ ] Chicken broth (p. 145)
- [ ] Frozen vegetables
- [ ] Bread: whole wheat, rye, sprout, kaiser buns, pita
- [ ] Fish fillets
- [ ] Individually-portioned chicken

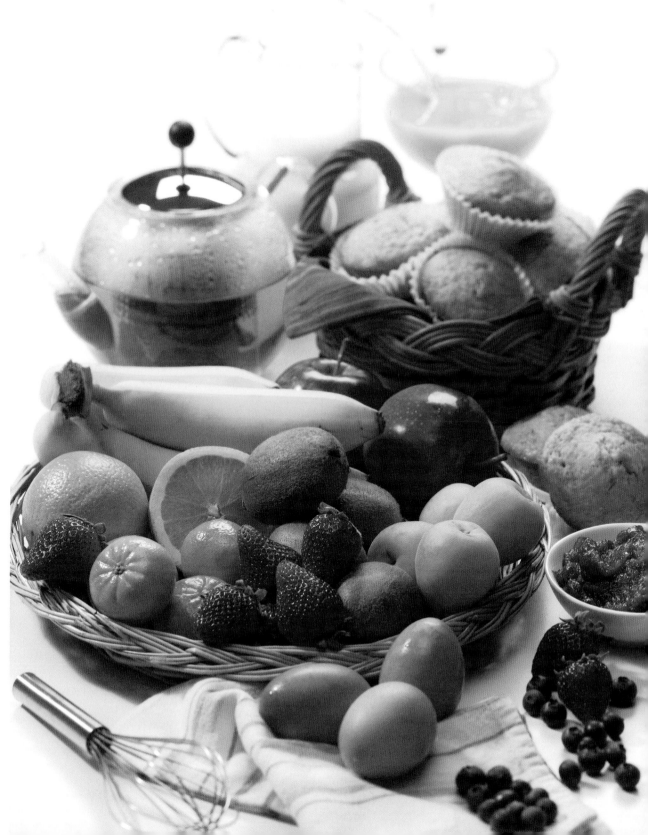

Breakfast

The perfect time to eat fruit

Dieticians, doctors, and nutritionists all agree that breakfast should be the most substantial meal of the day. Not necessarily the largest meal, but the most nutritious and with the most vitamins in order to give the body all of the nutrients it needs to function all day long. Nothing beats fruit to start the day on the right foot. Choose one that is listed in our top arthritis-fighting fruit line-up: pineapple, cantaloupe, orange and kiwi to name a few. If your mornings are rushed, pop fruit into the blender with other healthy foods for a quick on-the-go smoothie (see liquid breakfast recipe on page 137 for inspiration). Here are some other energizing and tasty ideas to kick-start your day.

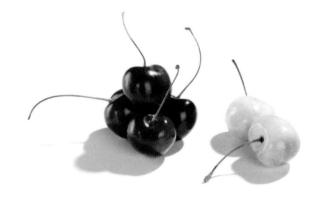

Breakfast

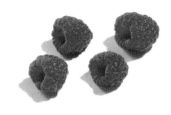

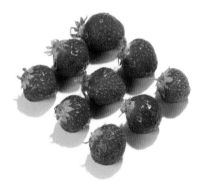

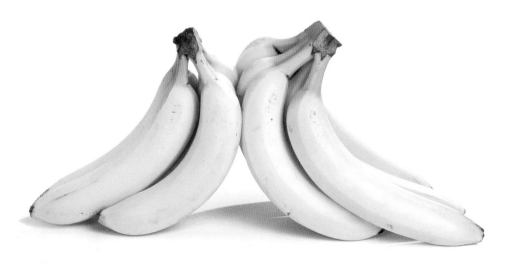

Kiwi compote with tea and ginger

Being a lazy cook, I prefer making preserves in small quantities to avoid sterilizing jars. If you find store-bought jams too sweet, you will like this recipe: it uses honey, is low in calories and is easy to make.

Ingredients (yields 1 ½ cup)

1 cup boiling water
1 green tea bag
3 medium-sized kiwis, peeled and sliced
20 dried apricot slivers, diced
2 tbsp raisins
4 cloves
2 cardamom pods, hulled
4 slices candied ginger
Juice and grated zest of one orange
3 tbsp honey

Preparation

❚ Steep tea for 5 minutes in boiling water.
❚ Pour tea in a small saucepan and add kiwis, apricots, raisins, clove, cardamom seeds and ginger. Bring to a boil and let simmer 20 minutes, uncovered.
❚ Pour orange juice, orange zest and honey on the fruit mixture and simmer 10 more minutes to thicken. Serve warm or cold.

Clementine and turmeric sauce

Delicious on toast, this sauce is also good as a frosting on cakes and squares.

Ingredients (yields ¾ cup)

1 tbsp non-hydrogenated margarine
2 clementines, peeled, sectioned and diced
1 tbsp honey
1 tbsp ginger marmalade
1 tsp turmeric
1 tsp cornstarch
½ cup orange juice

Preparation

❚ In a small saucepan, melt margarine and sauté clementine. Add honey, marmalade and turmeric; cook 2 minutes while stirring.
❚ Dissolve cornstarch in some of the orange juice, add to the fruit. Pour in remaining juice.
❚ Bring to a boil and let simmer until it thickens.
❚ Serve sauce warm as a compote or to garnish a dessert such as carrot cake (p. 265).

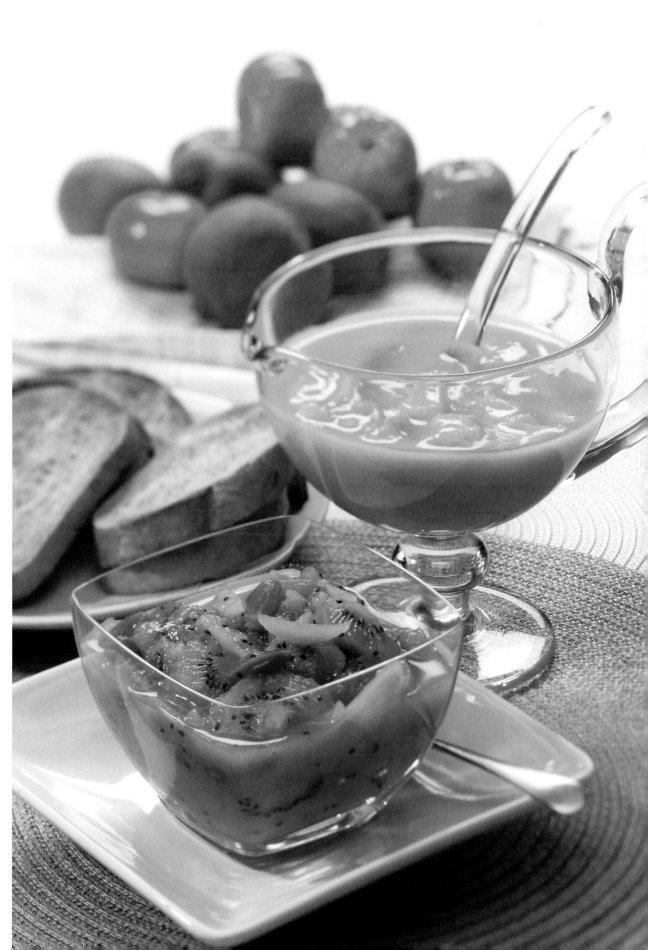

Orange and ginger muffins

Take the time to measure your dry ingredients the night before and these muffins will be a cinch to make the next morning.

Ingredients (12 muffins)

2 cups whole wheat pastry flour

1 ½ tsp baking powder

½ tsp salt

1 tbsp orange zest, grated

4 slices of candied ginger (or fresh), finely chopped

2 eggs

⅓ cup canola oil

½ cup brown sugar, firmly packed

2 tbsp orange marmalade

¾ cup vanilla soy milk

Preparation

▮ Preheat oven to 375°F.

▮ In a large bowl, combine flour, baking powder, salt, orange zest and ginger. Set aside.

▮ In another bowl, beat the eggs with the oil, brown sugar, marmalade and soy milk.

▮ Stir in dry ingredients and blend just enough to moisten dough.

▮ Spoon batter into oiled muffin tin (or line tin with paper cups).

▮ Bake 18 to 20 minutes or until toothpick inserted in the center comes out clean.

▮ Let cool 5 minutes before removing from tin.

Tip

▮ If you want to serve these muffins warm for breakfast, measure dry ingredients the night before. As soon as you wake up, you can continue the recipe from where it says to beat the eggs.

Quick green tea jam

This jam is fool-proof and quick to make. Dried fruit is quite sweet as it is so you don't have to add sugar. If the fruit you are using is not sweet enough, add a few teaspoons of honey to the tea. Delicious on toast!

Ingredients (one 6-ounce jar)

½ cup dried cranberries

½ cup dried apricots

½ cup dried strawberries

¼ tsp cinnamon

2 whole cloves

1 knob of fresh ginger, peeled

1 cup green tea

1 tsp orange zest, grated

Preparation

▮ In a small saucepan, combine cranberries, apricots and strawberries. Add cinnamon, cloves and ginger. Pour in the freshly brewed tea. Cook 20 minutes on very low heat. Remove ginger and cloves and let cool to lukewarm. Put through a food mill or purée in a blender or food processor. Add the orange zest, spoon into jars and keep refrigerated.

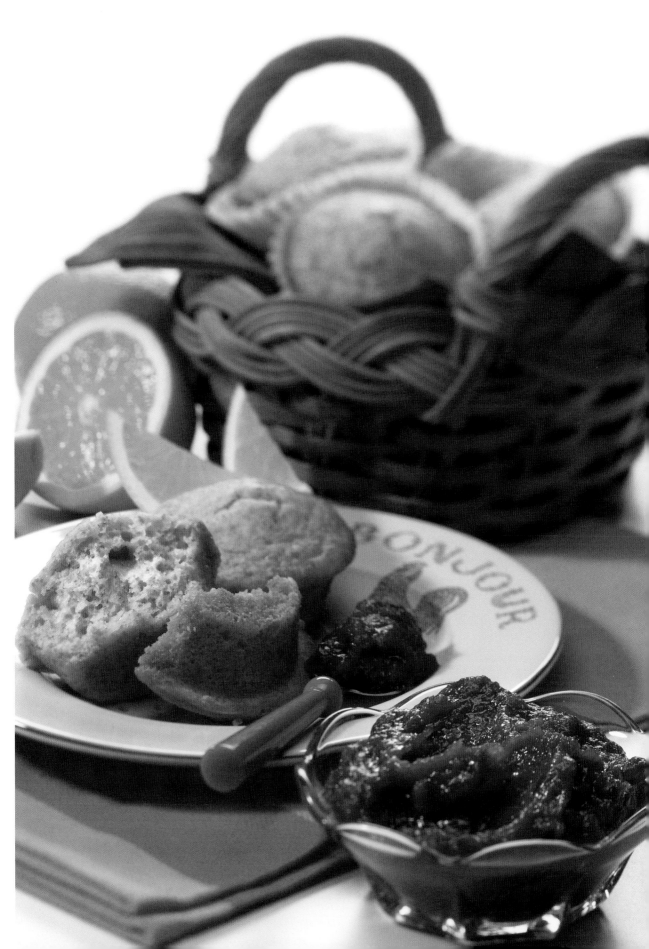

Rye crêpes

Sweeten this quick and easy crêpe recipe to your taste, but it is also delicious served as a savory entrée.

Ingredients (four and more)

1 ½ cups rye flour
1 ¾ cups unsweetened soy milk
½ cup water
2 large eggs
2 tbsp oil or non-hydrogenated margarine
½ tsp salt

Gourmet entrée version

▌ Try these crêpes as a side to your main dish by making savory versions with asparagus and goat cheese, or sweet pepper, tomato and pesto.

Preparation

▌ In a bowl, whisk all ingredients together. Set aside.

▌ In a frying pan, heat oil or margarine and pour in ¼ cup of the batter, spreading it out to form a round, thin crêpe.

▌ Cook 1 minute or until golden. Flip over with a spatula and cook the other side for 30 seconds. Transfer to a plate and cover with a cloth.

▌ Repeat until all the batter is used up. Serve with jam, marmalade or honey.

Honeydew melon and strawberry milkshake

This delectable beverage is a frothy blend of beta-carotein, protein and calcium that makes a perfect snack.

Ingredients for two

Half a honeydew melon, cut in pieces
½ cup vanilla soy milk
6 strawberries, fresh or frozen

Preparation

▌ Combine all ingredients in and serve.

Banana clementine smoothie

This tasty drink is a good alternative to commercial orange juice.

Ingredients for four

1 cup vanilla soy milk
1 ripe banana, cut in pieces
2 clementines, peeled and sectioned

Preparation

▌ Combine all ingredients in a blender, blend and serve.

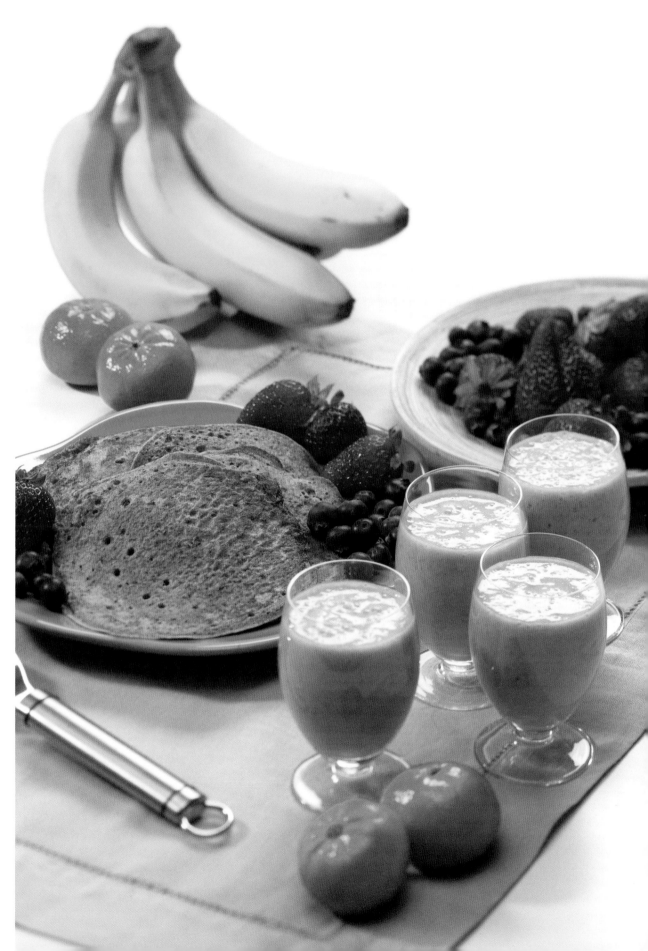

Cocoa pancakes with quick pear compote

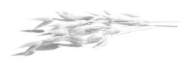

These pancakes are a tasty treat that you will want to serve for dessert. They can be made ahead of time and served cold or slightly reheated in the microwave.

Ingredients for two
(about 8 small pancakes)

1 egg, beaten
1 tbsp raw sugar
2 tbsp unsweetened cocoa
½ cup vanilla soy milk
⅓ cup whole wheat pastry flour
2 tbsp clementine juice
1 tbsp canola oil
½ tsp orange zest, grated
Non-hydrogenated margarine for cooking

Preparation

▌ Whisk together eggs, sugar and cocoa a few minutes until light and frothy. Add milk, flour, clementine juice, oil and orange zest. Refrigerate at least one hour (or overnight) before making pancakes.

▌ In a nonstick frying pan, heat oil at medium heat and melt margarine. Pour approximately ⅛ cup of batter. Cook until pancake center appears dry, turn over delicately and cook a few seconds longer. Repeat until batter is all used up. Stack pancakes on a plate putting a sheet of wax paper in between each one.

Pear compote

2 tbsp brown sugar
2 tbsp non-hydrogenated margarine
2 tbsp clementine juice
A few drops of vanilla extract
2 pears, cubed

Preparation

▌ In a saucepan, bring to boil brown sugar, margarine and clementine juice. Add pear cubes and let simmer 15 minutes then mash the pear with a fork. Add vanilla extract and serve warm or cold, on pancakes or on toast.

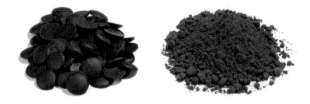

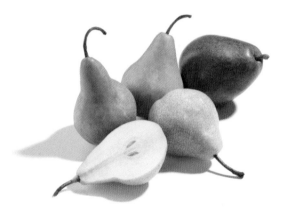

Liquid breakfast

For those of you who don't have time to sit at the breakfast table, this drink will keep you going until lunchtime.

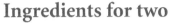

Ingredients for two

½ cup plain yogurt
½ cup plain soy milk
½ cup orange juice
1 tsp honey, or add more to taste
1 tsp ground flaxseed
6 almonds

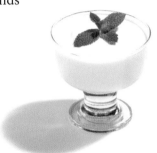

Add your favorite fruit to this mix:
- Half a mango, peeled and cubed
- Half a ripe banana, sliced; or 2 kiwis
- Half a pear, washed and cubed
- Half an apple, washed and cubed
- ½ cup blueberries (fresh or frozen)
- ½ cup strawberries (fresh or frozen)
- ½ cup pineapple, cubed

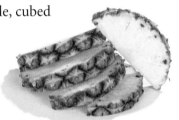

Honey and almond flakes

Use this recipe as a base to inspire your own cereal mix. All you need to do is add grain flakes such as rye, buckwheat, wheat, spelt; seeds such as sunflower, pumpkin, flax; nuts such as pecans, hazelnuts, pinenuts.

Ingredients (10 servings)

¼ cup canola or olive oil
¼ cup honey
3 cups regular rolled oats
½ cup sunflower seeds
¼ cup sesame seeds
½ cup almonds, slivered

Preparation

- Preheat oven to 350°F.
- In a small bowl, heat oil slightly in microwave (approx. 30 seconds).
- In a large oven-proof baking dish, combine rolled oats, almonds, sunflower and sesame seeds. Bake 20 minutes, mixing at half time. Cool and store in fridge in an airtight container. Serve with soy milk.

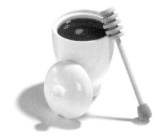

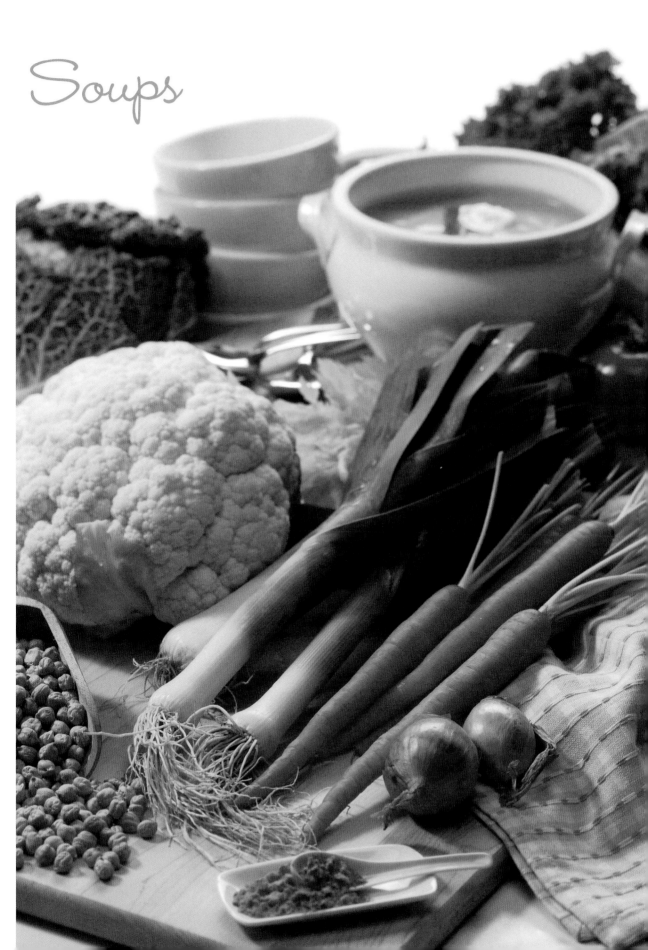

Soups

A great way to eat vegetables

For generations our mothers and grandmothers would use soup as a remedy for many ailments such as colds and indigestion, and to strenghten the weak and frail. Today soup still provides comfort and warmth. Preparing my chicken broth recipe requires little time and is well worth the extra effort after making a roast chicken meal (page 222). On page 144 you will find a vegetable broth recipe for a lighter soup base. No matter which broth recipe you choose, all you need to do is add any foods you have on hand to transform them into soups for a light lunch, a comforting pick-me-up or a meal that will stick to your ribs. Brimming with nutrition, the soups you prepare with these broths will benefit everyone in the family, even those that turn their noses up at vegetables. They are easy to make, easy to digest, incredibly versatile, and they offer a huge number of posibilities; they should feature front and center in your arthritis fighting diet.

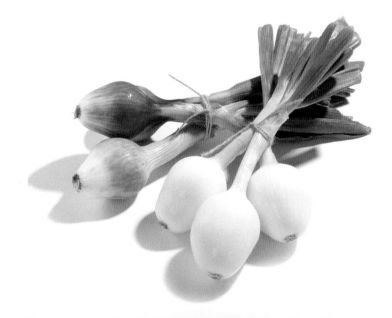

Soups

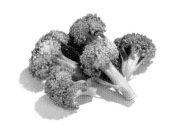

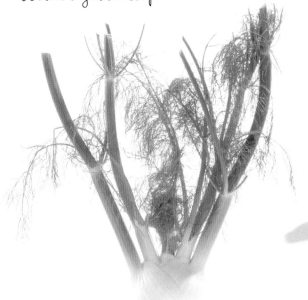

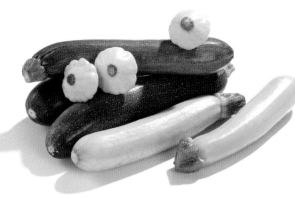

Carrot and ginger soup

The aromas in this simple soup are irresistible. You will surprise and delight your guests with the exotic perfume of cumin and coriander.

Ingredients (4 servings)

2 tbsp olive oil
4 medium carrots, peeled and sliced
2 medium zucchinis, peeled and sliced
1 small clove of garlic, finely minced
1 tsp fresh ginger, finely minced
1 tsp turmeric
1 tsp of the following spices: cumin, coriander, chili pepper flakes and ground fennel seeds
3 cups chicken broth (p. 145)
Salt and pepper to taste
2 tbsp cilantro, minced (to garnish)

Preparation

▌ In a saucepan, heat oil and sauté carrots and zucchinis 2 to 3 minutes. Add garlic, ginger, turmeric, spice mix and stir to blend well.
▌ Add broth, salt and pepper. Cover and bring to a boil. Lower heat and simmer 20 minutes.
▌ Cool, adjust seasoning, purée in blender or food processor and reheat. Garnish with cilantro and serve.

Gourmet version

▌ Reduce broth quantity to 2 cups for cooking and add 1 cup of coconut milk after puréeing.

Kale soup

Those who don't like cabbage will appreciate the lighter taste of kale; it is similar to rapini and is cooked like spinach.

Ingredients (6 servings)

3 tbsp olive oil
2 onions, chopped
3 cloves of garlic, finely chopped
2 10-oz cans chicken broth adding twice their volume in water, or 5 cups of homemade chicken broth (p. 145)
12 kale leaves, finely minced
1 15-oz can chickpeas, rinsed and drained
2 tbsp lemon juice
1 tsp lemon zest, grated

Preparation

▌ In a saucepan, heat oil and sauté onions. Add garlic, cover and cook 5 minutes over very low heat. Add broth, kale, chickpeas and lemon juice.
▌ Cover and bring to a boil. Add salt and pepper to taste. Lower heat and simmer 20 minutes, covered.
▌ Cool, purée in blender or food processor. Return to pot, adjust seasoning, add lemon zest. Reheat and serve.

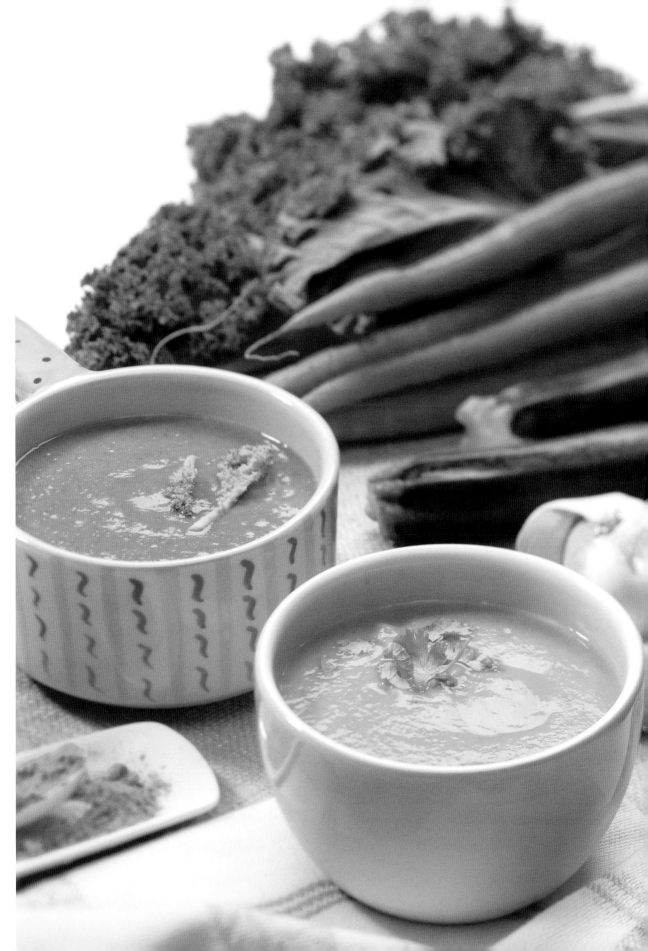

Homemade vegetable broth

This broth contains a bounty of nutrient-rich ingredients that will add flavor and nutritional value to your soups and stews. You can also switch it up by replacing the classic herb mix (thyme, basil, oregano, chervil) with an exotic blend of cumin, fennel, curry, chili pepper, star anise and coriander.

Ingredients

2 tbsp olive oil
2 onions, quartered (or 2 leeks, sliced)
2 carrots, sliced
1 parsnip, cubed
4 celery stalks with leaves, coarsely chopped
1 clove of garlic
12 cups water
2 bay leaves
1 tbsp herbs of choice
Salt and pepper to taste

Preparation

▌ In a stockpot, heat oil and sauté onions, carrots, parsnip, celery and garlic for 10 minutes. Add water, herbs and seasoning, cover and bring to a boil. Lower heat and simmer 1 hour, covered.
▌ Strain broth and discard vegetables.
▌ Store in fridge or divide in containers and freeze.

Green pea soup

Another easy soup to make and this one offers a velvety, palate-pleasing texture.

Ingredients (4 servings)

2 tbsp olive oil
1 large onion, chopped
1 small fennel bulb, chopped (about 1 cup)
3 medium zucchinis, peeled and cut in large pieces
1 clove of garlic
1 tsp curry powder
1 tsp turmeric
1 cup frozen green peas
3 cups vegetable broth or chicken broth (p. 144-145)
Salt and pepper to taste

Preparation

▌ In a saucepan, cook onions in oil until limp but not colored.
▌ Add fennel, zucchini, garlic, spices, peas and broth. Cover, bring to a boil, lower heat and cook 20 minutes over low heat, covered.
▌ Cool, add salt and pepper to taste and purée in blender or food processor. Reheat and serve.

Gourmet version

▌ Cut back ½ cup of broth and replace it with ½ cup of coconut milk after puréeing. Garnish with cilantro leaves.

Homemade chicken broth

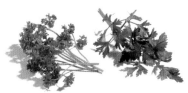

This broth is as tasty as it is affordable because you make it with the leftover chicken carcass from last night's dinner. Once the meat is gone, the bones and remaining scraps can be transformed into the perfect base for quick sauces and soups.

Ingredients (yields 6 cups or more)

Leftover roast chicken carcass (or from any other poultry), including cooking juices or sauce, skin, bones and any innards except the liver.

1 onion

1 carrot, brushed clean

1 celery stalk with leaves

1 clove of garlic, peeled

1 knob of ginger, peeled

1 tbsp tomato paste

1 sprig of parsley

1 bay leaf

1 tsp of various herbs (thyme, basil, oregano, chervil)

Water to cover the carcass

Salt and pepper to taste

Preparation

▌ Put all the chicken parts and juices in a stock-pot.

▌ Add remaining ingredients and enough water to cover (about 10 cups.)

▌ Bring to a boil, season to taste, lower heat and simmer at least 2 hours, covered.

▌ Cool completely (this will take all night if made in the evening), then strain.

▌ The broth will keep for many days in the fridge, covered in its fat. Before using, remove the congealed fat.

▌ Remove the fat before freezing, where it will keep for up to 6 months.

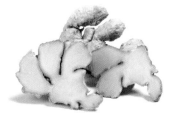

Poultry broth

All manner of poultry can be used to make flavorful broths: turkey, duck, pheasant, guinea hen, goose, quail, and many more.

Minute soup

This broth is a quick-fix in case of unexpected dinner guests; just add a bit of couscous, sliced mushrooms, parsley, carrot matchsticks, and a bit of tomato paste or sauce. Bring to a boil. Enjoy a delicious soup ready in less than 5 minutes.

Creamy cauliflower soup

This soup will seduce even those who don't usually like cauliflower. If you don't like the taste of curry powder, replace it with fresh or dried herbs.

Ingredients (4 servings or more)

2 tbsp olive oil
1 leek, finely minced
1 clove of garlic, finely chopped
1 small cauliflower, in florets
2 small zucchinis, peeled and cut in pieces
2 ½ cups chicken broth (p. 145)
2 tsp curry powder
1 tsp turmeric
½ tsp celery seeds
1 cup unsweetened soy milk
Salt and pepper to taste
2 tbsp parsley, chopped

Preparation

- In a saucepan, heat oil and cook leek over medium-low heat until limp but not colored.
- Add garlic, cauliflower florets, zucchini, broth, curry powder, turmeric and celery seeds.
- Cover and bring to a boil. Lower heat and simmer for 20 minutes or until cauliflower is tender.
- Cool, purée in blender or food processor and add soy milk. Salt and pepper to taste. This soup is delicious hot or cold. Garnish with parsley and serve.

Switch it up

- Feel free to replace soy milk with cow's or goat's milk, or coconut milk.

Tomato and chickpea soup

Inspired by a Syrian recipe, this spicy soup is one of my favorite staples in the winter.

Ingredients (4 servings)

1 tbsp olive oil
1 onion, chopped
2 cloves of garlic, chopped
1 cup canned tomatoes
1 19-oz can of chickpeas, rinsed and drained
2 cups chicken broth (p. 145)
1 tsp mint flakes
¼ tsp chili pepper flakes
½ tsp lemon zest, grated
1 tbsp lemon juice
Salt and pepper

Preparation

- In a saucepan, heat oil and lightly brown onions. Add garlic, cook for 2 minute. Add tomatoes, chickpeas, broth, mint and chili pepper flakes. Bring to a boil, lower heat and simmer 20 minutes. Purée with a hand mixer, add lemon zest and lemon juice, season to taste.

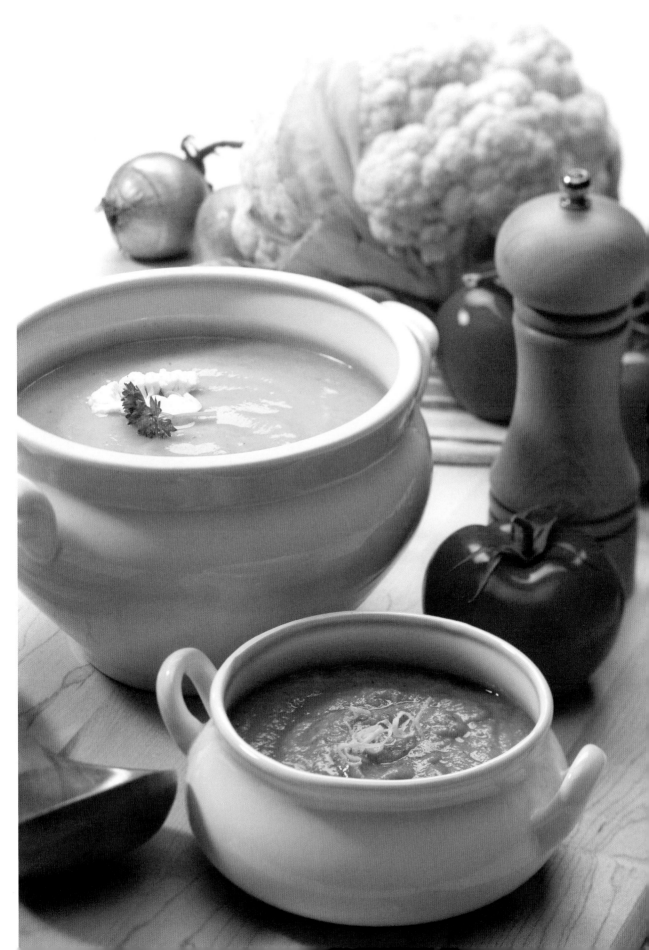

Quick minestrone

This thick and comforting soup goes well with a light meal or a salad. It is my go-to soup because I always have the ingredients on hand in the fridge and the pantry.

Ingredients (6 servings)

2 tbsp olive oil
1 large onion, chopped
1 clove of garlic, finely chopped
2 carrots, diced
1 thick slice of turnip, diced
1 small parsnip
1 celery stalk, diced
2 tbsp tomato paste
4 cups water
¼ cup soup pasta
1 19-oz can white kidney beans, rinsed
   and drained
1 to 2 cups chicken broth (p. 145)
Dried herbs (or fresh, in season), sage, thyme,
   oregano, marjoram and others
½ cup chopped parsley
Salt and pepper to taste

Preparation

▌ In a large saucepan, heat oil and lightly brown onion. Add garlic, carrot, turnip, parsnip, celery, tomato paste and water; cover and bring to a boil.

▌ Lower heat and simmer 15 minutes.

▌ Bring back up to a boil and add pasta, kidney beans and herbs. Cook 15 minutes, uncovered.

▌ Season to taste, add fresh parsley and serve.

Gourmet touch

▌ Add 1 tsp of pesto (p. 251) to each serving.

Tip

▌ I'm sure you've figured out that all vegetables are interchangeable in this recipe, which welcomes any leftovers you may want to use up.

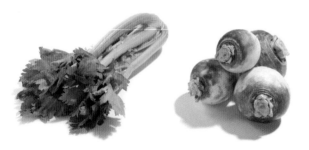

Hooray for leftovers!

▌ This rule of thumb is good for all soups: don't hesitate to combine any small portions of leftover soup together. Just add a bit of broth, maybe some quick-cook couscous, and voilà, a new recipe!

Fish soup in a flash

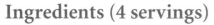

Quick to prepare, this soup will appeal even to those who aren't so fond of fish, thanks to the flavors of carrot and zucchini.

Ingredients (4 servings)

2 tbsp olive oil
1 dry shallot, finely chopped
2 small carrots, diced
2 zucchinis, cubed
1 clove of garlic, finely chopped
½ tsp pepper sauce
3 cups water or fish broth
1 tbsp tomato paste
8-oz fillet of fish (turbot or sole)
¼ cup white wine
Salt and pepper to taste
Toasted croutons

Preparation

▌ In a saucepan, heat oil and sauté shallot, carrot and zucchini over low heat.

▌ Add garlic, pepper sauce, water or fish broth and tomato paste. Bring to a boil, lower heat and simmer 15 minutes.

▌ Add fish and white wine, bring back to a boil, lower heat and let cook for 5 more minutes.

▌ Season to taste, blend with a hand mixer or food processor and reheat.

▌ Serve with croutons and garnish each serving with 1 tbsp of parmesan.

Cold cucumber soup

Inspired by Mediterranean cuisine, this refreshing soup requires no cooking and is perfect for the sunny hot days of summer.

Ingredients (4 servings)

5 Lebanese cucumbers, washed and unpeeled
¼ cup leek whites (or green onions), chopped
20 mint leaves
1 cup chicken broth (p. 145)
1 cup unsweetened soy milk
Salt and pepper to taste
Mint leaves for garnish

Preparation

▌ In a blender or food processor, combine cucumber, leek or green onion, mint, broth and soy milk; blend.

▌ Add salt and pepper, adjust seasoning and refrigerate at least one hour before serving.

▌ Garnish with mint leaves.

Gourmet touch

▌ For an occasional indulgence, add 1 tbsp of 15% table cream to each serving.

Spinach and white kidney bean soup

Nutritious and full of fiber, this quick and easy soup is ideal for arthritis sufferers.

Ingredients (4-6 servings)

2 tbsp oil
1 onion, chopped
2 cloves of garlic, finely chopped
2 cups spinach leaves, washed and trimmed, or half of a 10-oz package of frozen spinach
¼ tsp nutmeg
1 19-oz can white kidney beans, rinsed and drained
3 ½ cups chicken broth (p. 145)
1 tsp lemon juice
1 tsp lemon zest, grated

Preparation

▌ In a large saucepan, heat oil and lightly brown onion. Add garlic, spinach, nutmeg, kidney beans, broth, salt and pepper.

▌ Cover and bring to a boil. Lower heat and simmer 15 minutes.

▌ Blend with a hand mixer, add lemon juice and lemon zest; serve.

Celery soup with turmeric

Two essential vegetables that should always be on hand, celery and zucchini come together beautifully in this simple and delicious soup.

Ingredients (4 servings)

2 tbsp olive oil
2 cups celery, diced
1 leek, chopped
1 clove of garlic, finely chopped
1 tsp turmeric
1 zucchini, unpeeled and cubed
1 tsp fennel seeds
½ tsp pepper sauce
2 ½ cups chicken broth (p. 145)
Salt and pepper to taste

Preparation

▌ In a saucepan, heat oil and sauté celery and leek for 5 minutes; add garlic, cook for 1 more minute. Add turmeric, zucchini cubes, fennel seeds, pepper sauce and broth. Season to taste, cover, bring to a boil.

▌ Lower heat and simmer 20 minutes or until celery is tender. Remove from heat and cool. Purée in blender or food processor and reheat before serving.

Gourmet touch

▌ Add oven-toasted hazelnuts or almonds (toast 5 to 10 minutes at 350°F).

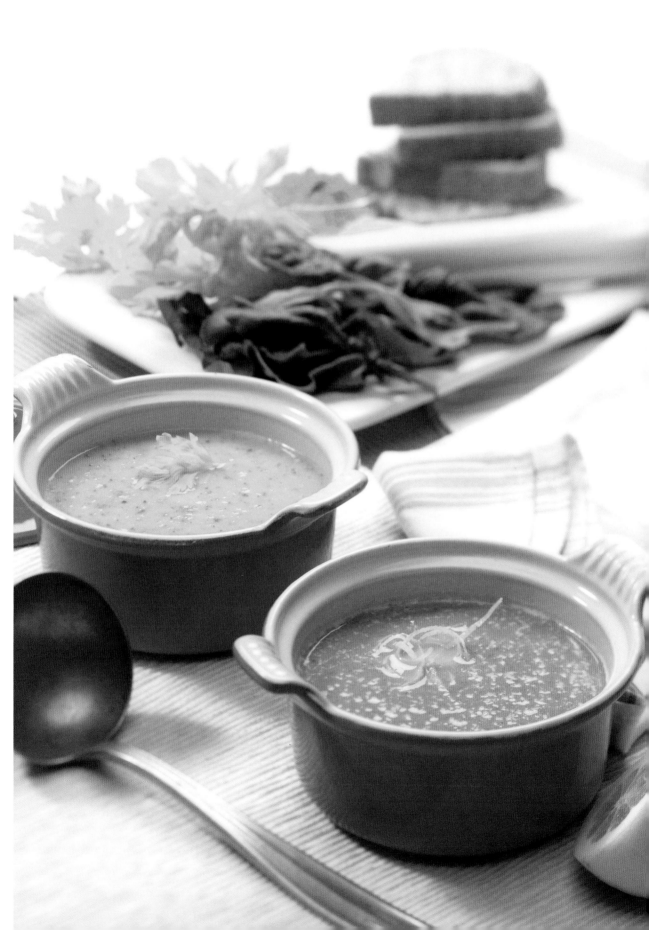

Squash and fennel soup

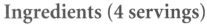

The mild taste of squash is enhanced by the bolder taste of fennel, which has an interesting aniseed taste, not unlike licorice.

Ingredients (4 servings)

1 small acorn squash, halved and seeded
1 tbsp oilve oil
½ tsp salted herbs (or any herb of your choice)
½ tsp sage
2 tbsp olive oil
1 leek, whites only, minced
1 yellow zucchini, unpeeled, cut in pieces
Half a fennel bulb, minced
½ tsp fennel seeds, ground
3 cups chicken broth (p. 145)
Salt and pepper to taste

Preparation

▌ Preheat oven to 350°F.
▌ Put the squash halves in a baking dish. Brush with olive oil, sprinkle with herbs and sage and bake 30 minutes or until tender. Remove flesh and set aside.
▌ In a saucepan, heat oil and lightly brown leek. Add fennel, squash, zucchini, fennel seeds, broth, salt and pepper. Cover, bring to a boil, lower heat and simmer 20 minutes.
▌ Cool and purée with mixer.
▌ Reheat and serve.

Broccoli soup

Broccoli goes well with many different vegetables. I love it paired with aniseed-tasting fennel. This recipe is a good base for you to transform according to your whims and the content of your fridge.

Ingredients (4 servings and more)

2 tbsp olive oil
1 small onion, chopped
2 zucchinis, peeled and cut in pieces
2 cloves of garlic
2 cups of broccoli florets
1 small fennel bulb, chopped
4 cups chicken broth (p. 145)
½ tsp celery seeds
Salt and pepper to taste

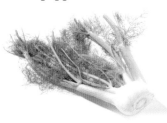

Preparation

▌ In a saucepan, heat oil and sauté onion and zucchini pieces. Add garlic, broccoli florets, chopped fennel and broth. Season to taste.
▌ Cover and bring to a boil, lower heat and simmer 20 minutes.
▌ Cool and blend with a mixer.

Switch it up

▌ Replace half of the broccoli with cauliflower florets since they are a perfect pairing.
▌ Replace zucchini with potato for a soup that has a starchier texture, but is just as delicious.

Winter vegetable soup

This soup is loaded with vegetables and perfect to eat with nice crusty bread. You can intensify its flavors by adding a spoonful of pesto in each bowl.

Ingredients (6 servings or more)

2 tbsp olive oil
1 large onion, chopped
2 cloves of garlic, chopped
6 cups chicken or vegetable broth
   (pp. 144 and 145)
3 tbsp pot barley
2 tbsp tomato paste
2 carrots, diced
½ cup rutabaga, diced
1 cup cabbage, finely minced
¼ cup fresh parsley, chopped
1 tsp dried herbs (sage, thyme, marjoram,
   savory)
Salt and pepper to taste

Preparation

▌ In a saucepan, heat oil and cook onions for 3 minutes until limp but not colored. Add garlic, broth, barley, tomato paste, carrot and rutabaga. Season, cover, bring to a boil, lower heat and simmer 20 minutes.

▌ Add the cabbage and simmer 15 minutes more, until vegetables and barley are tender.

Meal version

▌ Replace tomato paste with one can of whole tomatoes and add one can of chickpeas.
As with all soups, this will keep for 6 months in the freezer.

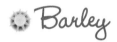 **Barley**

The best kind of barley to buy from a nutritional standpoint is definitely pot barley; it has a higher content of fiber, mineral salts, and thiamine.

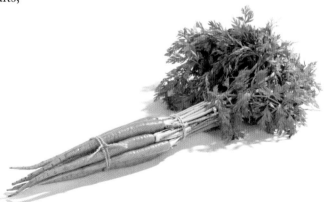

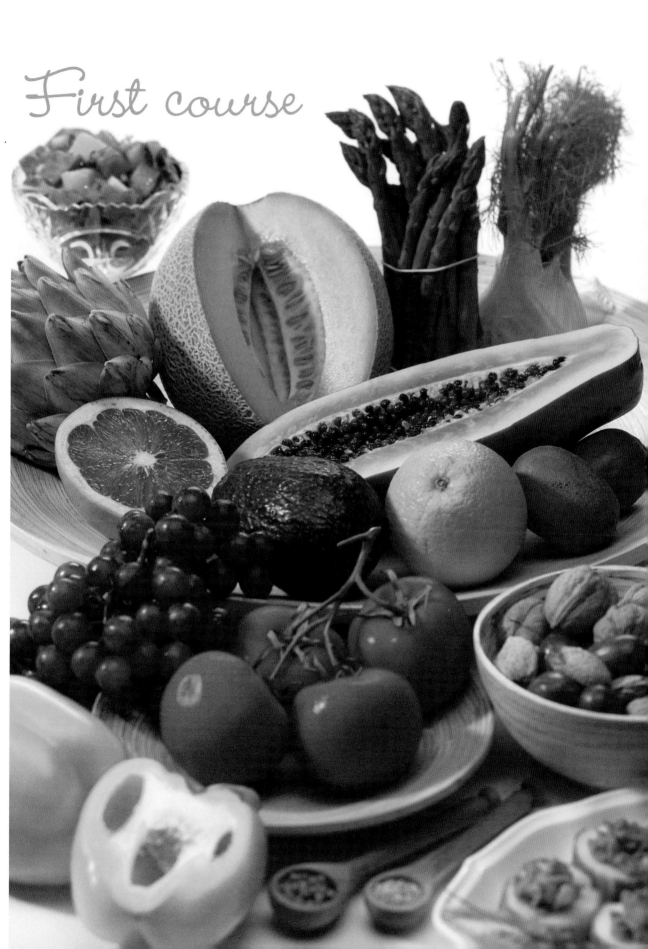

First course

An invitation to enjoy eating

The first course is meant to entice your tastebuds and whet your appetite without filling you up; it is an invitation to enjoy eating if you will. It should prepare your senses and stimulate your curiosity to discover the flavors still to come. Combinations made with fruits and vegetables are perfect as a first course. They offer freshness, tastes, and textures that complement each other beautifully as well as serve up a multitude of nutritional therapeutic benefits with each delectable bite. Aromatic herbs, orange zest, and lemon zest add extra zing to the mix, enhancing flavors. If the simple platter of crudités I suggest you start every meal with is not sophisticated enough, try these light and tasty dishes that require very little time and effort. Enjoy!

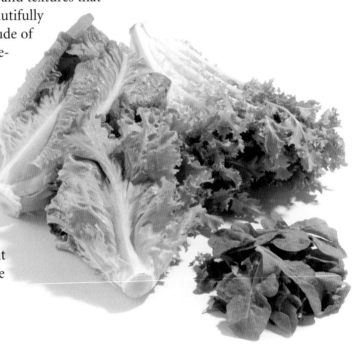

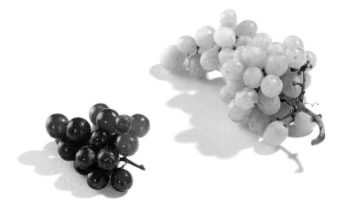

First course

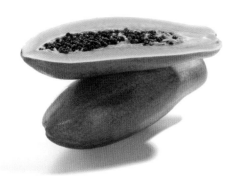

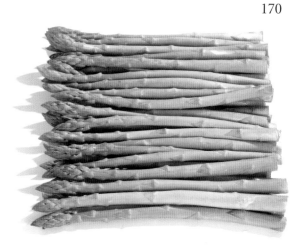

Orange flavored asparagus with pecans

Oven-baked asparagus infused with the aroma of orange make a light and elegant first course.

Ingredients (4 servings)

1 ½ lbs fresh asparagus, washed and trimmed
2 tbsp oil
2 tbsp honey
2 tbsp orange juice
1 tsp orange zest, grated
¼ cup pecans, coarsely chopped
Salt and pepper to taste
Mixed lettuce leaves

Preparation

▮ Preheat oven to 375°F.
▮ Spread asparagus out on a lightly oiled baking sheet. Set aside.
▮ In a small bowl, combine oil, honey, orange juice and orange zest; pour half of this mixture on the asparagus. Add salt and pepper and bake 7 to 8 minutes.
▮ Meanwhile, add the pecans to the remaining liquid mixture. When the asparagus are ready to come out of the oven, cover with the nut and liquid mixture and bake for another 7 to 8 minutes.
▮ Serve on a bed of lettuce.

Cantaloupe and grape salad with ginger

This refreshing salad is a happy mix of arthritis-busting ingredients.

Ingredients (4 servings)

1 cantaloupe, spooned out in bite-size balls
20 red seedless grapes, halved
3 cups baby spinach

Honey ginger vinaigrette
1 tbsp fresh ginger, grated
1 tsp Dijon mustard
1 tbsp honey
1 tsp sesame oil
¼ cup canola oil
Salt and pepper to taste

Preparation

▮ In a salad bowl, combine melon balls, grapes and baby spinach.
▮ In a small bowl, prepare the ginger dressing by whisking together ginger, mustard, honey, sesame oil and canola oil. Season to taste.
▮ Pour dressing on salad, mix well and serve.

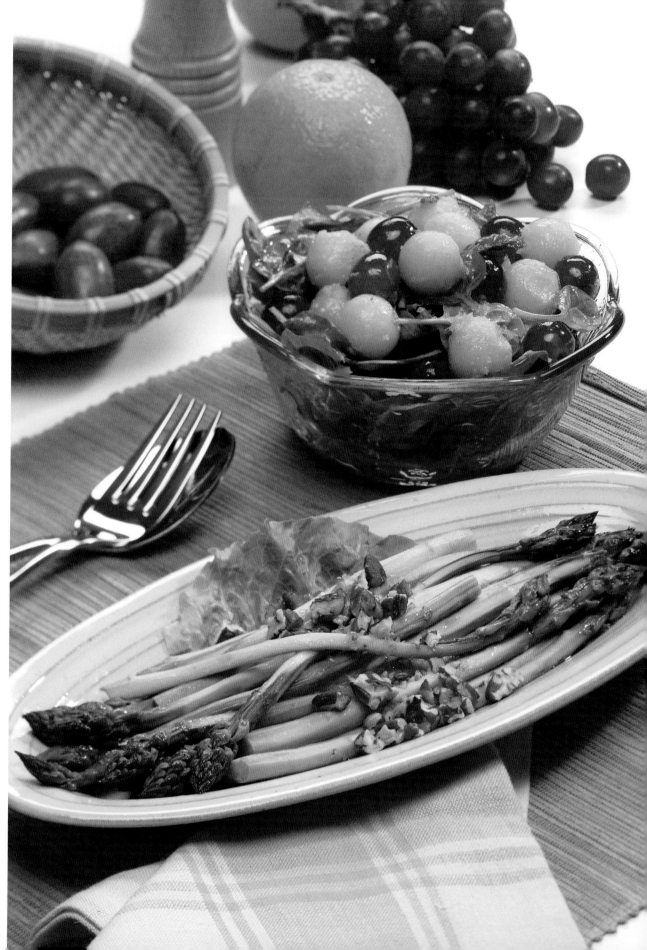

Stuffed avocados scented with lime and curry

You will love this delicious and nourishing first course, perfect before a light meal.

Ingredients (4 servings)

2 ripe avocados
7.5 ounce can of sockeye salmon
6 to 8 tbsp plain yogurt
2 tbsp light mayonnaise (or 1 tsp tahini)
¼ cup fresh chives or parsley, chopped
Zest of half a lime, grated
½ tsp curry powder
¼ tsp turmeric
Salt and pepper to taste
Lettuce or spinach leaves

Preparation

▌ Make the stuffing by draining and flaking the salmon and combining with the mayonnaise or tahini, parsley or chives, lime zest, curry powder and turmeric. Add salt and pepper to taste.

▌ Cut the avocados in two, remove pit and stuff each half with salmon mixture.

▌ Serve on a bed of lettuce or spinach.

Clementine and carrot salad with sage

Quick and easy to make, and low in calories, this sunny salad will brighten up your winter meals.

Ingredients (4 servings)

4 clementines, peeled, sectioned and chopped
4 endives, separated and cut in three
4 green onions, chopped
1 cup carrots, grated
¼ cup fresh parsley, chopped
¼ cup sesame seeds

Sage vinaigrette
½ tsp ground sage
½ tsp fennel seeds, ground
1 tbsp cider vinegar
1 tsp honey
1 tsp orange zest, grated
3 tbsp olive oil
Salt and pepper to taste

Preparation

▌ In a salad bowl, combine clementine, endive, green onion, carrot, parsley and sesame seeds.

▌ In a small bowl, whisk vinaigrette ingredients together.

▌ Pour on the salad, mix well and serve.

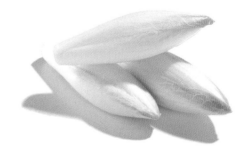

Salmon imperial triangles

A new twist on an Asian classic, these tasty bites are made with the same dough squares as imperial rolls but are baked in the oven for less fat and fewer calories than their fried counterparts.

Ingredients (12 triangles)

1 tbsp canola oil
1 dry shallot, minced
1 small clove of garlic, minced
12 mushrooms, finely chopped
7.5 ounce can of sockeye salmon
½ cup slivered almonds, coarsely chopped
¼ cup fresh parsley, chopped
4 tbsp parmesan
Salt and pepper to taste
Egg white to seal
12 squares imperial roll dough measuring
   5.5 inches, thawed
2 tbsp olive oil

Preparation

▌ Preheat oven to 400°F.
▌ In a frying pan, lightly brown shallot, add garlic and mushrooms and cook over low heat until cooking juices evaporate. Cool and set aside.
▌ In a bowl, combine drained salmon, almonds, parsley and parmesan; add mushroom mixture and season.
▌ Lay down a square of dough and brush edges with egg white. Drop 2 tbsp of filling on one diagonal half; fold over opposite corner to form a triangle. Pinch edges to seal. Repeat with all dough squares.
▌ Place triangles on a lightly-oiled or parchment paper-lined baking sheet. Brush each triangle lightly with oil. Bake 15 minutes or until golden.

Waste not, want not!

▌ Leftover filling? Add it to soup or pasta. Leftover dough squares will keep for two days in the fridge, wrapped in plastic wrap.

Gourmet variation with pistachio

1 tbsp non-hydrogenated margarine
1 dry shallot, minced
2 cloves of garlic, minced
16 mushrooms, chopped
½ cup pistachios, shelled and coarsely
   chopped
Salt and pepper to taste

Preparation

▌ In a frying pan, melt margarine and sauté shallot and garlic. Add mushrooms and cook until their cooking juices evaporate.
▌ Add pistachios, salt and pepper.
▌ Continue with the rest of the triangle preparation instructions.

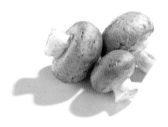

Black bean salad

Intensely colorful, this salad is perfect for a light lunch and is a guaranteed hit at a buffet, served with dips and vegetarian terrines.

Ingredients (4 servings)

1 tbsp lemon juice
1 small clove of garlic, minced
3 tbsp olive oil
2 tbsp fresh parsley, chopped
½ tsp spice mix (coriander, cumin, ground fennel seeds, mint)
19 ounce can of black beans, rinsed and drained
Half of a red onion, finely chopped
Half of a sweet yellow pepper, diced
Half of a Lebanese cucumber, diced
1 ripe tomato, diced
12 stuffed green olives, chopped

Preparation

▌ In a salad bowl, combine lemon juice and garlic; add olive oil, parsley and spices, blend well.
▌ Add black beans, onion, yellow pepper, cucumber, tomato and olives.
▌ Mix well, refrigerate 1 hour before serving.

Omega-3 rich variation

▌ Add a can of sardines or salmon and flake with a fork for a complete meal.

Winter tabbouleh with sundried tomatoes

Tomatoes are harder to find and less flavorful in the winter–they're more expensive too! Try this winterized version of a classic featuring artichokes and olives.

Ingredients (4-6 servings)

1 cup couscous (wheat semolina)
1 tbsp olive oil
4 tbsp sundried tomato, finely chopped
1 cup boiling water
5 tbsp olive oil
2 tbsp lemon juice
1 tbsp dried mint
1 tsp dried oregano
½ cup fresh parsley, chopped
4 canned artichoke hearts, chopped
16 black olives, pitted and chopped
Salt and pepper to taste

Preparation

▌ In a salad bowl, combine couscous, one tbsp olive oil, dried tomatoes and boiling water; mix well. Cover and let stand 10 minutes. Fluff with a fork and cool.
▌ In a small bowl, combine the remaining oil, lemon juice, mint and oregano. Pour onto couscous. Mix well, add parsley, artichoke hearts and olive pieces. Season to taste, keeping in mind that black olives are salty. Serve warm or cold.

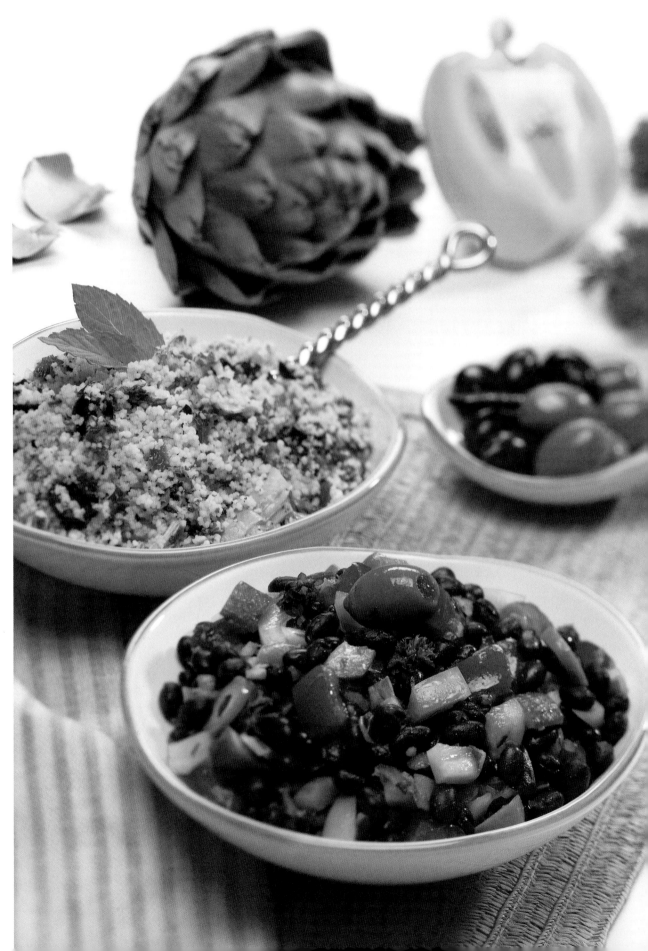

Buckwheat and mushroom terrine

This delicious meatless terrine is an excellent alternative to pâtés and cold cuts. Its consistency is similar to head cheese.

Ingredients (6 servings and more)

1 tbsp olive oil
1 dry shallot, minced
1 small clove of garlic, minced
½ cup mushrooms, chopped
½ cup white buckwheat, washed and drained
¼ cup regular rolled oats
1 ¾ cups chicken broth (p. 145)
1 tsp tamari sauce
½ tsp ground coriander
½ tsp fennel seeds, ground
¼ tsp ground clove
Salt and pepper to taste
1 tbsp agar-agar flakes (available in health
   food stores)

Preparation

▮ In a saucepan, heat oil and lightly brown shallot. Add garlic and mushrooms and sauté for 2 minutes.

▮ Add buckwheat, oats, chicken broth, tamari sauce and spices; bring to a boil, lower heat and simmer 15 minutes.

▮ Season, add agar-agar, blend delicately and simmer for 2 more minutes.

▮ Pour into lightly-oiled bread pan, cool before refrigerating.

▮ Serve on bread or crackers.

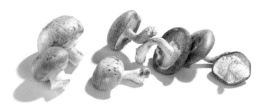

❁ Buckwheat

Buckwheat contains substances that are thought to be cancer-inhibiting. It is rich in rutin, a glycoside that improves blood circulation and lowers blood pressure. Buckwheat is gluten-free and highly recommended for people with gluten intolerances, celiac disease, and other digestive ailments. It is sold in health food stores.

❁ Oats

Contrary to other cereals, oats do not lose their bran and germ after being processed, which is where most nutrients are found in the grain. Oats' high concentration of fibre–particularly in the gelatinous substance that sticks to the pot when making oatmeal–make it the food of choice for people trying to lose weight.

Carrot and beet salad

Quick and easy to make, this tasty salad is perfect for feeding unexpected guests. You can replace the arugula with any leafy greens such as spinach.

Ingredients (4 servings)

3 medium carrots, grated
14 ounce can of whole beets, diced
1 apple, grated and drizzled with lemon juice to keep from turning brown
4 tbsp olive oil
2 tbsp clementine juice
1 tsp Dijon mustard
½ tsp turmeric
½ tsp dried mint
½ tsp orange zest, grated
1 ½ cups baby arugula, washed and spun dry

Preparation

▮ In a salad bowl, combine carrot, beet and apple.
▮ In a small bowl, whisk oil, clementine juice and mustard premixed with turmeric, mint and orange zest.
▮ Pour this dressing on the carrot mixture and toss well. Add arugula, toss again and serve.

Fresh variation

▮ You can replace canned beets with fresh, raw, grated beets. They are just as tasty and even more nutritious.

Red cabbage salad

Colors and flavors together in perfect harmony.

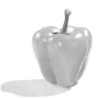

Ingredients (4 servings)

2 green onions, thinly sliced
1 sweet yellow pepper
1 tbsp balsamic vinegar
3 tbsp olive oil
¼ tsp cajun spice mix (p. 253)
Salt and pepper to taste
2 cups red cabbage, finely shredded
½ cup white kidney beans
¼ cup fresh parsley, chopped
12 black olives, pitted and chopped
1 tomato, chopped

Preparation

▮ In a small bowl, prepare vinaigrette by whisking together green onion, yellow pepper, vinegar, oil, cajun spices, salt and pepper.
▮ Pour vinaigrette on shredded cabbage and refrigerate one hour.
▮ Add white kidney beans, parsley, black olives and tomato. Serve.

Papaya, mango and kiwi salad infused with vanilla

Vanilla gives these fresh fruits a delightfully distinct flavor. Serving this salad with a meat dish will make it easier to digest.

Ingredients (4 servings)

3 cups of cubed fruit (papaya, mango, kiwi)
1 tsp vanilla extract
1 tbsp lemon juice
2 tbsp balsamic vinegar
2 tbsp walnut oil
2 tbsp canola oil
¼ tsp Chinese five-spice powder
¼ tsp hot pepper sauce
1 cup mixed lettuce leaves
4 tbsp pine nuts, dry-pan toasted
1 tbsp papaya seeds* (optional)

* *Papaya seeds give this salad a peppery taste.*

Preparation

▊ In a large bowl, whisk together dressing ingredients: vanilla, lemon juice, vinegar, oils, spices and hot pepper sauce. Add fruit, mix and refrigerate one hour.

▊ In pretty dessert cups, make a nest of greens, top with fruit mixture and garnish with pine nuts and papaya seeds. Serve.

Sweet variation

▊ Replace vinegar and oils with ¼ cup orange juice, omit hot pepper sauce and serve this salad for dessert.

Mackerel or sardine canapés

These quick and easy appetizers are finger-licking good.

Ingredients (15 canapés)

4 ounces mackerel fillets, or sardines packed in oil, drained
1 to 2 tbsp plain yogurt
1 small clove of garlic, minced
½ tsp curry powder
½ tsp turmeric
¼ tsp fennel seeds, ground
½ tsp lemon zest, grated
2 tbsp dill, chives or parsley
Endive leaves, cucumber or zucchini slices, or crackers to serve on
Salt and pepper to taste

Preparation

▊ In a small bowl, flake mackerel or sardines with a fork; combine with yogurt, garlic, curry, turmeric and fennel seeds. Refrigerate 30 minutes.

▊ Add lemon zest, herb of choice (dill, chives or parsley) and mix. Season to taste.

▊ Garnish endive leaves or spread on cucumber slices or crackers.

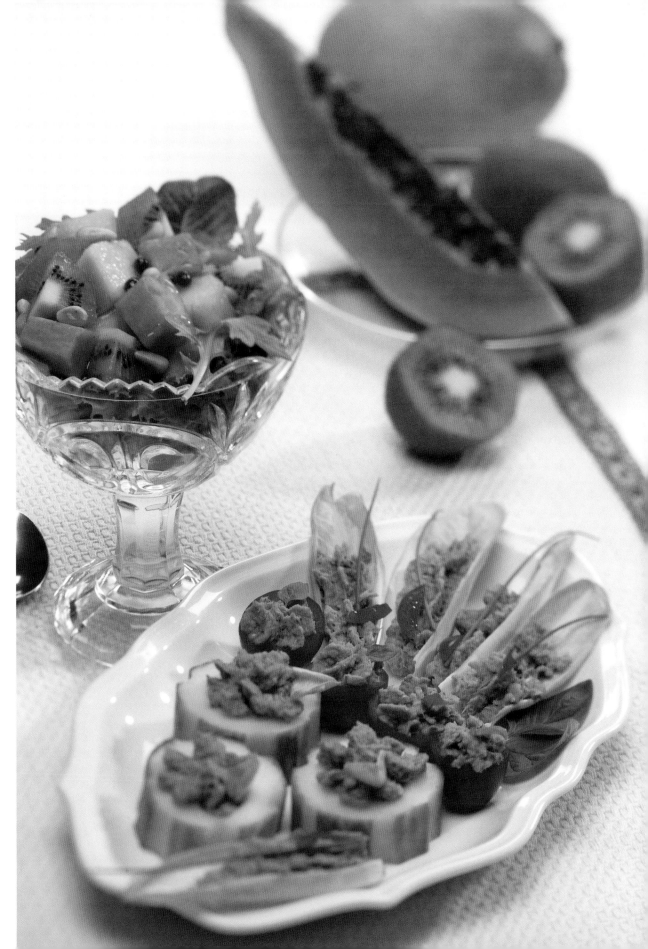

Melon and avocado salad

This omega-3 rich salad is a refreshing first course. The delicate taste of the melon is superb with the creaminess of the avocado.

Ingredients (4 servings)

2 endives, cut in three and separated
Half a honeydew melon, cut in pieces
1 ripe avocado, cut in pieces and drizzled with lemon juice
20 or so red grapes, halved
2 cups mixed lettuce leaves

Tahini dressing
1 tsp tahini
½ tsp lemon zest, grated
1 tsp tamari sauce
½ tsp sesame oil
2 tbsp olive oil
2 tbsp canola oil
Dash of hot pepper sauce
Salt and pepper to taste

Preparation

▌ In a salad bowl, combine endive, melon, avocado and grapes.

▌ In a small bowl, whisk together dressing ingredients. Season to taste and add to the fruit.

▌ Put lettuce in pretty dessert cups, top with fruit salad and serve.

Gourmet version

▌ For a perfect summer salad, replace grapes with fresh strawberries.

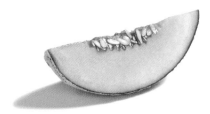

❁ Melon

Not only is melon delicious, but it is full of beneficial nutrients like antioxidant vitamin C and beta-carotein, which have a rust-proofing effect on joints.

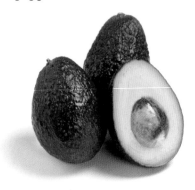

❁ Avocado

Avocado is rich in glutathione, an antioxydant capable of relieving joint pain. It is great for anyone looking to improve flexibility and mobility.

Asian style artichokes

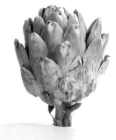

Fast and easy cooking in the microwave preserves all of the artichoke's properties. They are then dressed with a brightly-flavored Asian vinaigrette.

Ingredients (4 servings)

4 artichokes
Cold water

Vinaigrette
1 tsp tamari sauce
1 tsp rice vinegar
1 tsp sesame oil
2 green onions, minced
1 clove of garlic, minced
2 slices of fresh ginger, minced
¼ tsp hot pepper sauce
¼ cup canola oil
Pepper to taste

Preparation

- Trim artichokes, cut stems, remove small leaves at base, rinse in cold water.
- Place each into a ramequin with 2 tbsp of cold water.
- Cover each artichoke loosely with plastic wrap.
- Cook 12 to 15 minutes.*
- Meanwhile, whisk together vinaigrette ingredients. Pour vinaigrette over artichokes. Serve warm with bread.
- * *Cooking time for 1 artichoke: 5-7 minutes; 2 artichokes: 10-11 minutes; 3 artichokes: 12-15 minutes.*

Endive and fennel salad with apple

Anise-flavored fennel adds brightness to this French cuisine classic.

Ingredients (4 servings)

2 cups mixed lettuce leaves
4 small endives, cut and separated
1 cup fennel, finely slivered
1 dry shallot, minced
2 apples, peeled, diced and drizzled with lemon juice to keep from turning brown
4 thin slices of sweet yellow pepper, finely diced
⅓ cup hazelnuts, coarsely chopped

Yogurt vinaigrette
2 tsp honey
1 tsp Dijon mustard
½ tsp lemon zest, grated
½ tsp turmeric
½ cup plain yogurt
Salt and pepper to taste

Preparation

- Place lettuce leaves on four plates.
- In a salad bowl, whisk together vinaigrette ingredients.
- Add endive, fennel, shallot and apple.
- Mix well and spoon onto plates. Garnish with diced yellow pepper and hazelnuts. Serve.

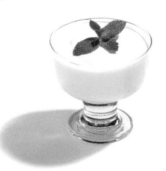

Mango and watercress salad

The sweetness of the mango is enhanced by this fragrant dressing. Don't forget that eating one or two mangos a week will help keep joint pain at bay as well as keep skin soft and supple.

Ingredients (4 servings)

1 mango, cubed
1 bunch of watercress, trimmed
1 cup of mixed lettuce leaves
4 endives, leaves separated and cut in three
2 tbsp sesame seeds

Asian vinaigrette

1 tsp tamari sauce
1 tsp rice vinegar
1 tsp sesame oil
2 green onions, minced
1 clove of garlic, minced
¼ tsp hot pepper sauce
¼ cup canola oil
Salt and pepper to taste

Preparation

▌ In a salad bowl, combine mango, watercress, lettuce leaves and endive. Toss gently.
▌ Whisk together vinaigrette ingredients, season lightly (tamari sauce is salty) and pour on salad. Sprinkle with sesame seeds, mix well and serve.

Grapefruit, avocado and fennel cup

This refreshing trio is a delightful way to brighten a winter meal. The acidity of the grapefruit is tempered by the creaminess of the avocado and livened by the crunch of the fennel.

Ingredients (4 servings)

1 pink grapefruit, peeled and sectioned
1 ripe avocado, cut in pieces and drizzled with
    lemon juice
1 small fennel bulb, thinly sliced
4 tbsp olive oil
1 tbsp lemon or lime juice
Zest of half a lemon (or lime), grated
½ tsp hot pepper sauce
Salt and pepper to taste
2 tbsp sesame seeds
Arugula leaves (or any other lettuce)

Preparation

▌ In a bowl, combine grapefruit, avocado and fennel.
▌ In a small bowl, whisk together oil, juice and zest of lemon or lime and hot pepper sauce. Season to taste.
▌ Pour dressing on grapefruit mixture.
▌ Serve in pretty dessert cups on a bed of greens and garnish with sesame seeds.

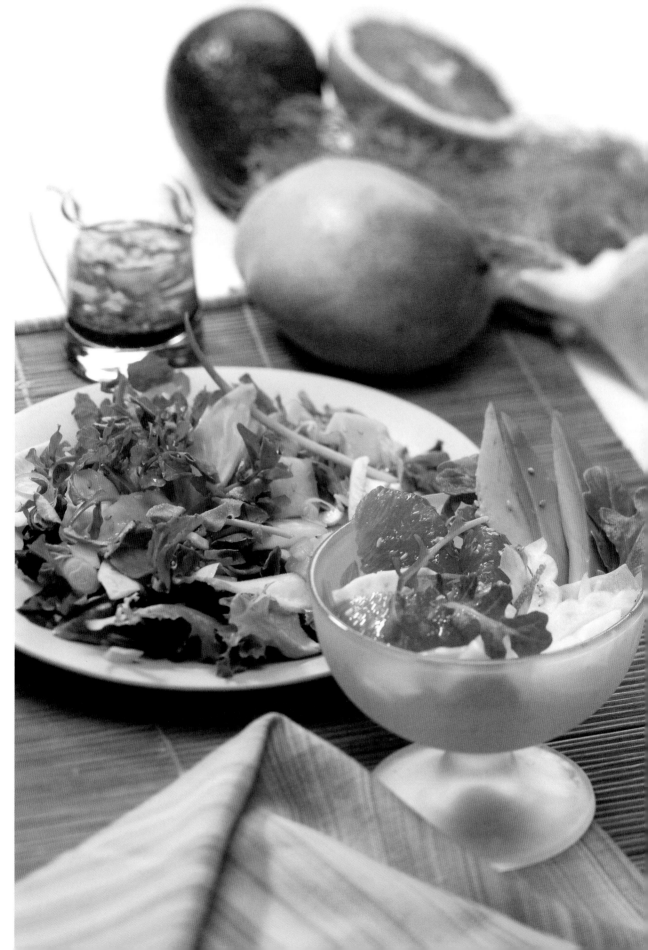

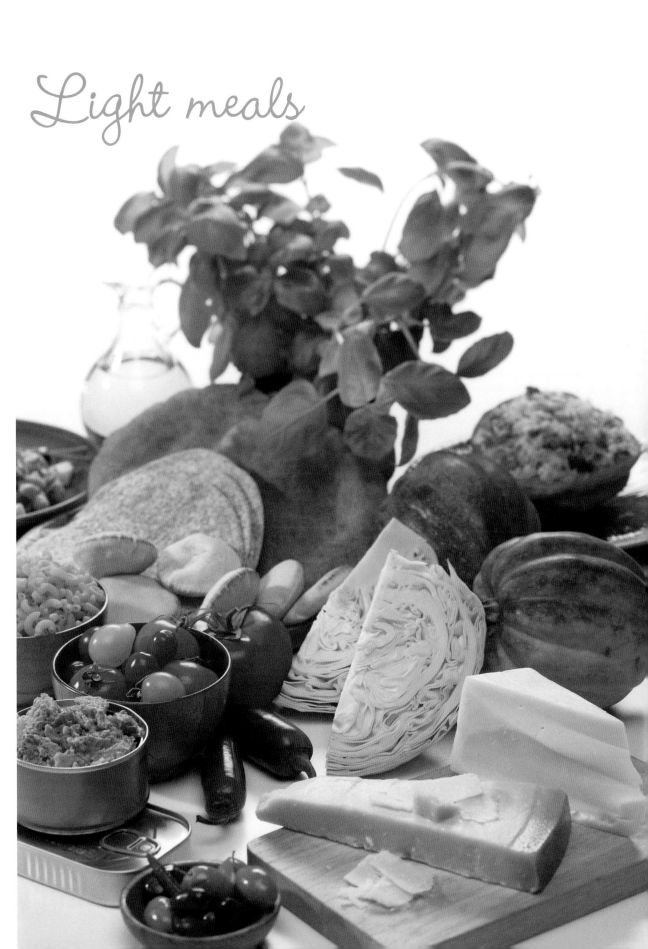

Light meals

Fast healthy food

I would like to propose some recipes for quick and easy meals. Like fastfood, they will nourish those in a rush; unlike fastfood, these are meatless dishes prepared with healthy ingredients. I want to prove that it is possible to replace convenient fastfood restaurant choices that are loaded with fat and sugar ,with light, nutritious, and delicious alternatives.

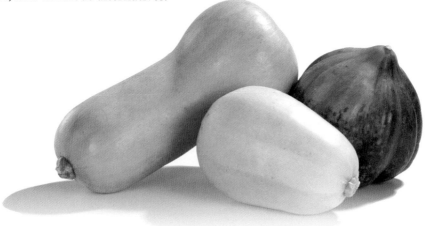

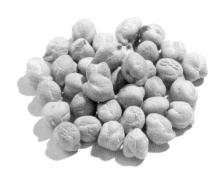

Light meals

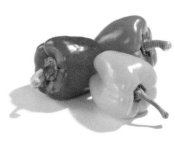

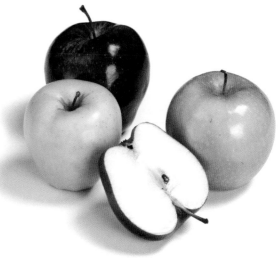

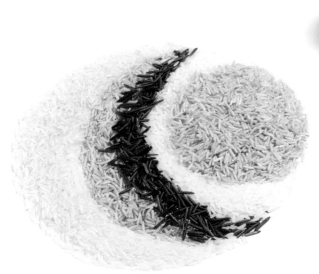

Express squash stuffed with salmon and rice, cooked in the microwave

*If you think squash takes a long time to cook, you have to try this recipe.
You will be pleasantly surprised by the fast and tasty results.*

Ingredients (2 servings)

1 small acorn squash, halved and seeded
4 tbsp water
Half a 7.5 ounce can of sockeye salmon,
   drained
1 cup cooked rice
1 dry shallot, or 2 green onions, chopped
A handful of diced low-fat cheese
¼ cup pine nuts or any other nut
¼ cup fresh parsley, chopped
Salt and pepper to taste

✴ Omega-3s

Mother Nature provides foods that have proven anti-inflammatory properties. They may
not be as strong as medicine, but they are safe
and highly recommended for arthritis sufferers because they relieve joint pain.

✴ Salmon

Rich in omega-3s, salmon has anti-inflammatory properties. It is also rich in vitamin D,
which is essential for bone health. It is one of
the fattiest of the oily fish, but it is still lower
in fat than red meat and its fat is healthy.
Canned salmon also has the advantage of not
losing its nutritional value.

Preparation

▮ In a microwave-safe Pyrex dish, place two
squash halves flesh side down. Add 4 tbsp
water and cover loosely with plastic wrap.

▮ Microwave on high for 8 minutes.

▮ Meanwhile, prepare stuffing. In a bowl, combine flaked salmon, rice, shallot or green
onion, cheese, nuts and parsley; mix well.
Season to taste and set aside.

▮ When squash is cooked, drain any remaining
water and stuff with salmon mixture.

▮ Reheat squash in microwave on high for
3 minutes.

▮ If desired, add a bit of cheese and melt in the
oven for 1 minute.

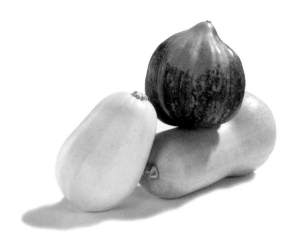

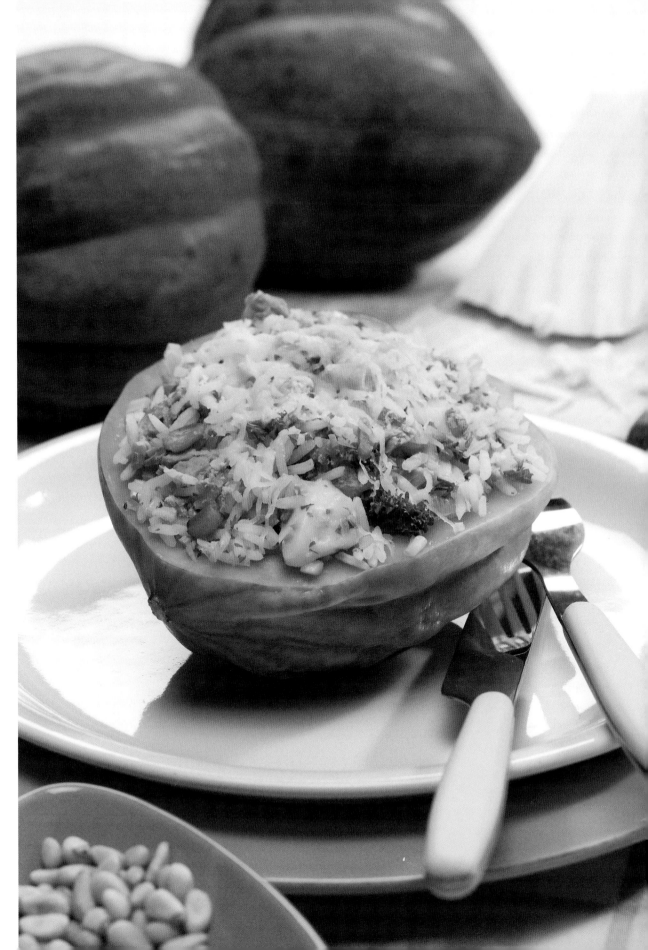

Mackerel fillet burgers

Prepared with canned fish, these burgers are quick to make and simply delicious.

Ingredients (4 servings)

2 cans (4.5 ounces each) mackerel fillets,
  finely chopped
2 eggs, beaten
1 ½ cups breadcrumbs, a little more if needed*
1 dry shallot, minced
2 tbsp parsley, chopped
1 tsp dried tarragon
1 tsp lemon zest, grated
1 tbsp olive oil or non-hydrogenated margarine
Salt and pepper to taste
4 kaiser rolls

* *Be creative! You can make breadcrumbs using nuts, crackers, or cereal seasoned with your favorite herbs and spices.*

Preparation

▮ In a bowl, combine eggs and fish. Add bread-crumbs, shallot, parsley, tarragon and lemon zest; mix well.
▮ Make 4 patties. If the mixture is too moist, add more breadcrumbs.
▮ In a frying pan, heat oil and brown patties, 3 minutes on each side.
▮ Put patties in the rolls and toast in a sandwich toaster.

Pizza with goat cheese and pesto

Another version of home-made pizza, this one is flavorful and dressed with mushrooms and pecans.

Ingredients (4 servings)

4 wheat tortillas, 9 inches in diameter
¾ cup mushrooms, finely chopped
½ cup pesto (p. 251)
¼ cup pecans, chopped
Half a red onion, thinly sliced
1 cup partially-skimmed mozzarella
½ cup goat cheese, diced
1 tbsp sesame seeds

Preparation

▮ Preheat oven to 450°F.
▮ Place tortillas on pizza pans or baking sheets.
▮ Combine mushrooms, pesto and pecans; spread out on tortillas.
▮ Cover with red onion slices, sprinkle with cheese pieces and sesame seeds.
▮ Bake 7 minutes.

Omega-3 variation

▮ Substitute pecans with canned sockeye salmon.

Tortilla cups with curried chicken

This is a fun way to use up leftover chicken. These tortilla cups would also be delicious filled with steamed vegetables, broccoli and cauliflower florets or even tofu cubes and legumes.

Ingredients (4 servings)

4 wheat tortillas, 10 inches in diameter and
  a bit of oil
1 tbsp olive oil
1 small red onion, chopped
Half a yellow sweet pepper, diced
1 medium carrot, diced
1 small clove of garlic, minced
1 tbsp non-hydrogenated margarine
3 tbsp flour
2 tsp curry powder
1 tsp turmeric
½ tsp orange zest, grated
¼ tsp hot pepper sauce
1 cup chicken broth (p. 145)
1 cup plain, unsweetened soy milk
2 cups cooked chicken, cubed
2 tbsp fresh cilantro, chopped
Salt and pepper to taste

Preparation

▮ Preheat oven to 375°F.

▮ To make cups: Fold tortillas into 4 lightly-oiled ramekins 4.5 inches in diameter, to resemble a flower. Sit a smaller 2.5-inch ramekin on top, making sure to oil the bottom first to prevent from sticking to the tortilla. Bake 10 minutes. Lower heat to 350oF and transfer tortilla cups to lowest grill to keep "petals" from burning. Bake 5 more minutes. Wait a few minutes before taking tortilla cups out of ramequins, set aside.

▮ In a saucepan, heat oil and sauté onion, yellow pepper, carrot and garlic over medium heat for 10 minutes or until carrots are cooked al dente. Add flour, curry powder, turmeric, orange zest and hot pepper sauce; cook 1 minute. Add broth, soy milk, cilantro, salt and pepper; cook gently until thickened. Add chicken and heat in sauce.

▮ Pour mixture into tortilla cups and bake 10 minutes in the oven.

✿ Turmeric

This spice is known not only for its distinct taste but also for its antioxidant and anti-inflammatory properties. It is used in many ways, from curry to food coloring–it gives mustard its bright yellow hue–and is highly recommended for arthritis sufferers.

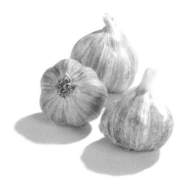

Black bean burritos

Mexican-inspired, these tasty tortilla roll-ups stuffed with black beans and fresh tomatoes are a quick and easy meal.

Ingredients (4 servings)

2 tsp olive oil
1 small onion (or shallot), chopped
1 small sweet yellow pepper, diced
2 cloves of garlic, minced
2 tomatoes, peeled, seeded, chopped and drained
2 tbsp cilantro, chopped
1 tbsp lime juice
1 tsp lime zest, grated
1 tsp chili seasoning (p. 253), or more to taste
Salt and pepper
19 ounce can black beans, rinsed and drained
4 wheat tortillas 10 inches in diameter
1 cup gruyère or cheddar cheese, grated

Preparation

▌ Preheat oven to 350°F.
▌ In a frying pan, heat oil and lightly brown onion or shallot, and yellow pepper. Add garlic, tomato, cilantro, lime juice and zest, chili seasoning and black beans. Bring to a boil and simmer 15 minutes, covered. Add salt and pepper to taste.
▌ Spoon a quarter of mixture into the middle of a tortilla. Gently roll up, hold together with a toothpick and place in a lightly-oiled baking dish. Repeat with each of the remaining tortillas.
▌ Sprinkle with grated cheese and bake 10 minutes or until cheese is melted.

Pasta salad with salmon

Canned salmon is incredibly versatile in making all sorts of delicious dishes. This salad is sure to please with a winning combination of salmon, nappa cabbage and arugula.

Ingredients (4 servings)

2 tbsp lemon juice
Zest of half a lemon, grated
4 tbsp olive oil
2 tbsp sesame seeds
4 tbsp fresh parsley, finely chopped
Salt and pepper to taste
1 cup nappa cabbage, finely shredded
2 cups short pasta, cooked
7.5 ounce can sockeye salmon, drained and flaked
12 black olives, pitted and finely chopped
1 cup arugula leaves

Preparation

▌ In a salad bowl, make vinaigrette by whisking together lemon juice, lemon zest, olive oil, sesame seeds, parsley, salt and pepper.
▌ Put cabbage in vinaigrette, then add pasta; mix well and refrigerate one hour.
▌ Add salmon, black olives and arugula, mix well and serve.

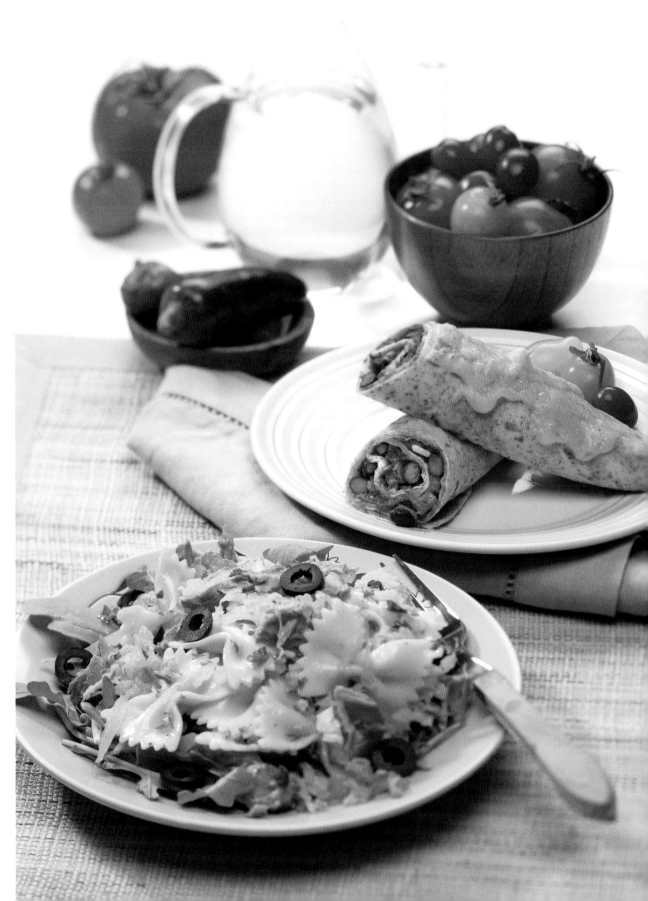

Chickpea croquettes

Thes croquettes are a great alternative to hamburgers for a nice, light lunch.

Ingredients (4 servings)

2 cups canned chickpeas, rinsed and drained
1 small red onion, chopped
¼ cup cilantro leaves, chopped
2 tbsp hazelnuts, ground
2 tbsp flaxseed, ground
2 tbsp fresh lemon juice
2 tbsp tahini
1 smalll clove of garlic, minced
1 tsp spice mix (mint, fennel, coriander, cumin)
Salt and pepper to taste
2 tbsp olive oil

Preparation

▌ In a food processor, combine chickpeas, onion, cilantro, hazelnut, flaxseed, lemon juice, tahini, garlic, spices, salt and pepper. Process until smooth. Shape into 4 croquettes.

▌ In a frying pan large enough for 4 croquettes, heat oil and brown them, about 3 minutes on each side.

▌ Serve with a sauce of your choice, such as tomato sauce (p. 250), or with a dip and oven-toasted pita triangles (p. 193).

Burger variation

▌ Put the croquettes in a kaiser roll and toast in a sandwich toaster.

Nut burgers

Here is yet another meatless burger alternative. This one is just as tasty thanks to sunflower seeds, zucchini and couscous.

Ingredients (4 servings)

1 cup unsalted sunflower seeds, ground
½ cup pecans or hazelnuts, ground
1 cup zucchini (or carrot), finely chopped
½ cup cooked couscous (or another cooked grain such as millet or rice)
2 tbsp plain yogurt
2 tbsp tahini
Salt and pepper to taste
1 tbsp non-hydrogenated margarine
4 kaiser rolls

Preparation

▌ In a bowl, combine all ingredients and shape into patties. If they are too moist, add couscous or nuts.

▌ In a frying pan, heat the margarine and brown patties, 3 minutes on each side just enough to warm them up.

▌ Put patties in kaiser rolls and toast 2 minutes in a sandwich toaster.

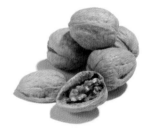

Cabbage and apple salad

A perfect union of flavor and nutrients, this antioxidant salad offers super protection against infection.

Ingredients (4 servings)

3 cups green cabbage, finely shredded
2 small carrots, grated
1 small shallot, minced
19 ounce can chickpeas, rinsed and drained
2 McIntosh or Empire apples, diced
3 tbsp fresh cilantro or parsley, finely chopped

Vinaigrette

2 tbsp cider vinegar
2 tsp honey
1 tsp curry powder
1 tsp turmeric
1 tsp ginger, minced
1 tsp orange zest, grated
6 tbsp olive oil
Salt and pepper to taste

Preparation

▌ In a salad bowl, whisk together vinaigrette ingredients. Season to taste.
▌ Add cabbage, carrot and shallot, mix well.
▌ Refrigerate one hour.
▌ Add apple, chickpeas, cilantro or parsley, mix well and serve.

Apple

Biting into an apple is pleasing and helpful at keeping the doctor away. Not only is it rich in vitamins and minerals, it also contains quercetin, an inflammation-busting antioxidant.

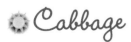

Cabbage

The list of ailments cured by cabbage over the centuries is impressive, if sometimes quirky. Its high concentration of carotenoids make it an invaluable ally in the prevention of joint degeneration and health problems related to aging.

Fresh tomato pizza

This pizza is as easy to make as it is good to eat. It can also be made with pita bread, cooked 12 to 15 minutes in a 400°F oven.

Ingredients (4 servings)

4 whole wheat tortillas, 9 inches in diameter
2 cups mozzarella or light cheese, grated
1 large sweet onion (red or white), thinly sliced
1 large sweet yellow pepper, seeded and thinly sliced
4 large tomatoes, thinly sliced
½ tsp dried oregano
2 tbsp fresh basil, chopped
12 to 15 black olives, pitted and chopped
4 tbsp parmesan
Salt and pepper to taste

Preparation

▌ Preheat oven to 450°F.
▌ Place tortillas on pizza pans or baking sheets. Spread each tortilla with cheese then onion and yellow pepper slices. Add tomato slices. Sprinkle with oregano, basil, olives and parmesan. Season to taste.
▌ Bake 7 minutes.

Gourmet variation

▌ This pizza is superb when fresh tomatoes are in season. It is even better if you brush a spoonful of pesto (p. 251) on each tortilla before adding garnishes.

Chicken and chickpea salad

This is a simple, nutritious, and delicious way to use up leftover roast chicken.

Ingredients (4 servings)

1 small red onion, diced
1 celery stalk, diced
1 zucchini, unpeeled and diced
19 ounce can chickpeas, rinsed and drained
1 ½ cups cooked chicken, diced
5 ounces feta cheese, diced
2 tbsp lemon juice
6 tbsp olive oil
1 tsp dried oregano
4 tbsp fresh chives or parsley, chopped
4 tbsp sweet red pepper, diced
Salt and pepper to taste

Preparation

▌ In a salad bowl, combine onion, celery, zucchini, chickpeas, cooked chicken and feta cheese.
▌ In a small bowl, whisk together lemon juice, olive oil and oregano. Season to taste and refrigerate for one hour before serving. Garnish with chives and diced red pepper.

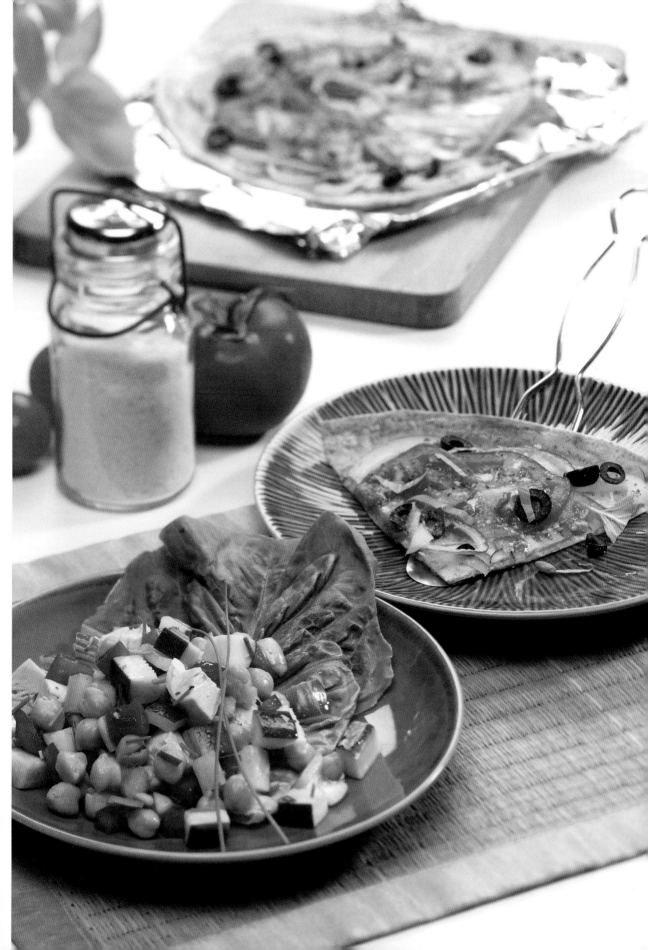

Meatless mains

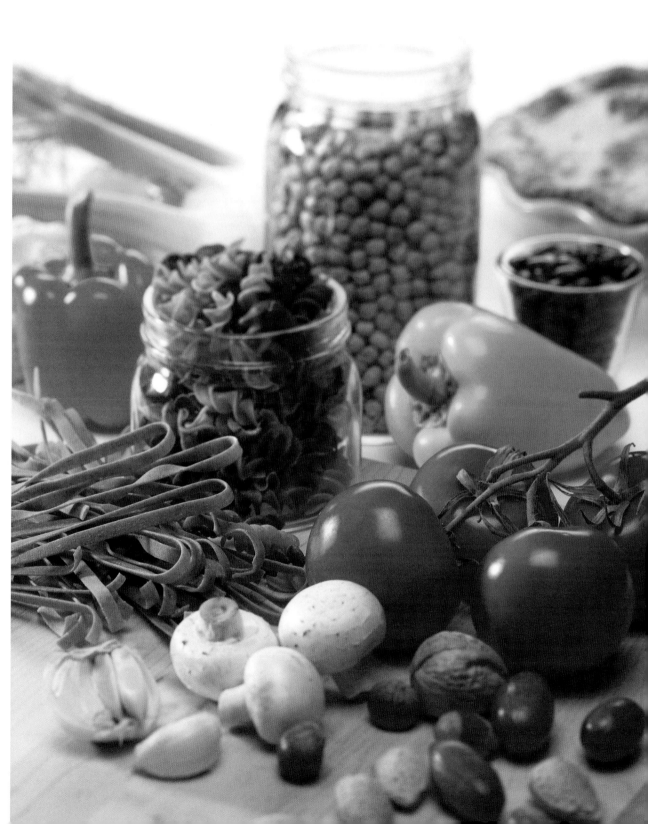

Reconciling what we want and what we need

Every good meal should offer what is best to satisfy both our cravings and our needs. By bringing out the best of vegetables with herbs, spices and a little help from fruit, veggies can shine as the stars of a healthy and satisfying meal.

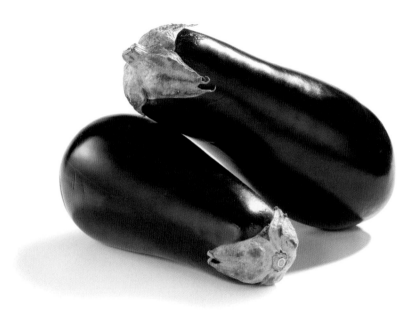

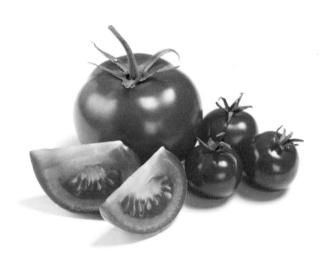

Meatless mains

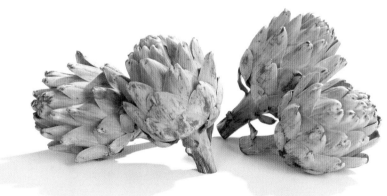

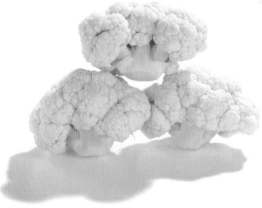

Fusilli with cauliflower and cherry tomatoes

A feast for the eyes and for the tastebuds, this pasta dish brings together an unusual pairing of vegetables.

Ingredients (4 servings)

12 ounces spinach fusilli
4 cups cauliflower florets
3 tbsp olive oil
8 anchovy fillets, soaked 5 minutes in water, drained and chopped
2 cloves of garlic, minced
¼ tsp chili flakes
¼ cup chicken broth (p. 145)
1 ½ cups cherry tomatoes, halved
¼ cup capers, rinsed and drained
¼ cup black olives, chopped
¼ cup pine nuts, oven-toasted
¼ cup parmesan, grated
¼ cup fresh parsley, chopped
Salt and pepper to taste

Preparation

▌ In a large pot of salted boiling water, cook pasta for 6 minutes, then add cauliflower florets and continue cooking 4 minutes until pasta is *al dente* and cauliflower is tender.

▌ Meanwhile, heat oil in a frying pan and sauté anchovy fillets, garlic and pepper flakes. Add broth, cherry tomatoes, capers and olives; continue cooking over medium heat.

▌ Drain cooked pasta and cauliflower and return to pot. Season to taste. Add tomato sauce and mix well. Add pine nuts, sprinkle with parmesan and parsley to serve.

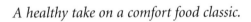

Macaroni casserole with mushrooms and cashews

A healthy take on a comfort food classic.

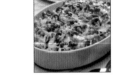

Ingredients (4 servings)

12 ounces macaroni
2 tbsp olive oil
8 ounces mushrooms, thinly sliced
1 ¾ cups tomato sauce (p. 250)
¼ cup fresh parsley, chopped
Salt and pepper to taste
¼ cup pimento-stuffed green olives rings
½ cup cashews
1 cup gruyère or cheddar, grated

Preparation

▌ Preheat oven to 400°F.

▌ In a large pot of salted boiling water, cook macaroni *al dente* according to the instructions on the package. Drain and pour in a baking dish, drizzle with olive oil.

▌ In a frying pan, heat 2 tbsp oil and sauté mushrooms for 5 minutes. Add tomato sauce and parsley, season and mix well. Sprinkle with olives and cashews, cover with cheese and bake 20 minutes. Serve with a vegetable salad.

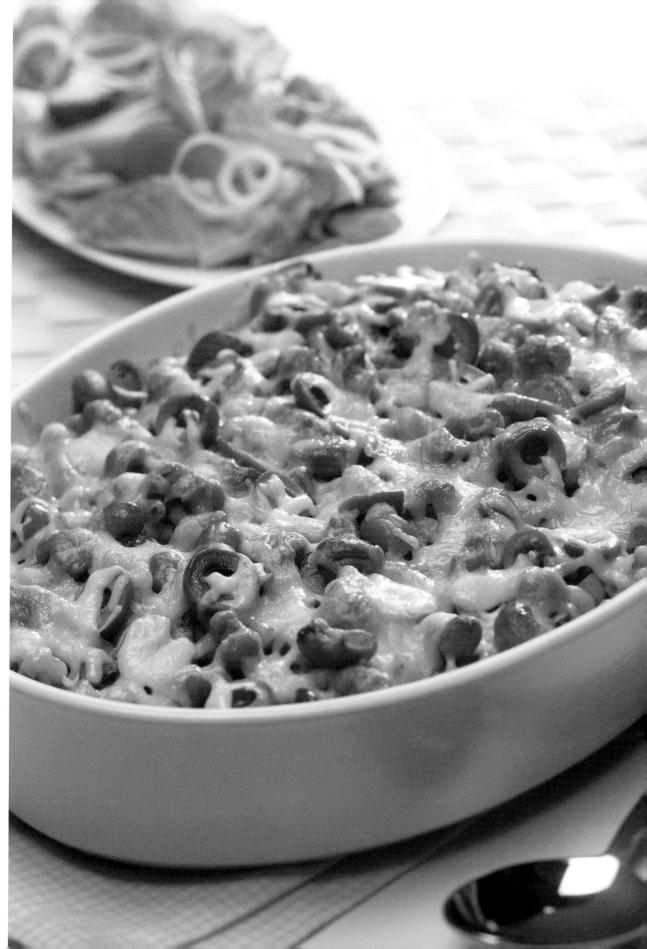

Meatless shepherd's pie

This version of shepherd's pie is healthier and just as flavorful as the meat version thanks to your favorite herbs and spices. For a sweeter approach, try substituting sweet potatoes for half of the regular potatoes.

Ingredient (4 servings)

4 yellow potatoes, peeled and cut in pieces
4 tbsp fresh parsley, chopped
1 tsp olive oil
2 tbsp olive oil
1 small onion, chopped
1 small clove of garlic, minced
19 ounce can brown lentils, rinsed and drained
½ cup chicken broth (p. 145)
1 tsp spice mix (cumin, coriander, mint, ground fennel)
19 ounce can of creamed corn
Salt and pepper to taste

Preparation

▌ Preheat oven to 350°F.
▌ In a small saucepan filled with salted water, cook potatoes for 20 minutes. Mash with parsley and one teaspoon of olive oil. Set aside.
▌ In a frying pan, lightly brown onions in oil. Add garlic, lentils, broth and spices; bring to a boil, simmer 20 minutes or so until liquid is absorbed.
▌ Pour into an 8-inch square baking dish, cover with creamed corn. Top with mashed potatoes. Bake 30 minutes or until hot.

Gourmet variation

▌ Add ½ cup chopped pistachios to the lentil mix.

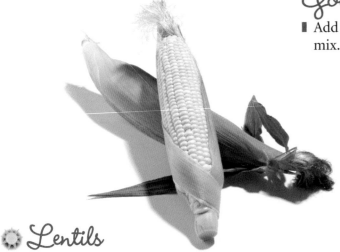

✿ Lentils

Eating legumes like lentils two to three times a week is a good way to increase fiber intake and help prevent cardiovascular disease and many types of cancer. And good news: canned lentils keep all of their nutritional value.

Lentil and fruit picadillo with golden pitas

This vegetarian version of a traditional Latin American dish is a great and tasty opportunity to replace meat with legumes.

Ingredients (4 to 6 servings)

2 tbsp olive oil
2 onions, chopped
2 cloves of garlic, minced
2 cans (19 ounces each) lentils, rinsed
    and drained
1 apple, peeled and cubed
¼ cup stuffed olives, chopped
6 tbsp raisins
½ tsp chili flakes
¼ tsp ground clove
2 ½ cups canned vegetable juice
Salt and pepper to taste
½ cup slivered almonds, oven-toasted
    (5-10 minutes at 350°F).

Preparation

▌ In a frying pan, heat oil and lightly brown onions. Add garlic, lentils, apple, olives, raisins, chili flakes, vegetable juice, salt and pepper. Cover, bring to a boil, lower heat and simmer 15 minutes. Uncover and simmer 15 more minutes or until liquid is completely evaporated. Sprinkle with almonds.

▌ Serve with spiced pitas (see recipe below).

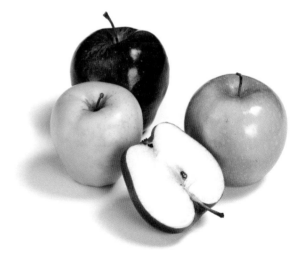

Golden pitas

Ingredients

4 pitas
2 tbsp olive oil
2 tsp herb and spice mix (cumin, paprika, coriander, fennel seeds, mint, chili flakes)

Preparation

▌ Preheat oven to 350°F.
▌ Combine spice mix and oil; brush on pita.
▌ Using kitchen shears, cut pita in triangles and bake 5 to 10 minutes until golden.

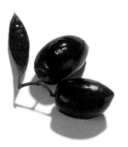

Short pasta with roasted vegetables

True Italian cuisine aficionados will love this simple but delicious dish that blends the light aniseed-perfumed fennel with the more potent flavors of sweet peppers, tomato and eggplant.

Ingredients (4 servings)

1 eggplant, cut in ½ inch pieces
1 sweet yellow pepper, cut in ½ inch pieces
1 fennel bulb, chopped
4 fresh, ripe tomatoes, quartered and sliced,
    or 6 canned tomatoes, drained and diced
3 cloves of garlic, minced
½ tsp chili flakes
Salt and pepper to taste
5 tbsp olive oil
2 tbsp olive oil
1 lb short pasta of your choice
Boiling, salted water to cook pasta

Preparation

▌ Preheat oven to 400°F.

▌ In a large bowl, combine eggplant , sweet pepper, fennel, tomato, garlic, chili flakes and 5 tablespoons of olive oil. Mix well. Spread out on a baking sheet lined with parchment paper or in an oiled roasting pan. Add salt and pepper.

▌ Bake 20 to 30 minutes until vegetables are tender and lightly roasted, stirring every 10 minutes.

▌ Meanwhile, cook pasta in boiling salted water according to cooking time indicated on package. Drain, return to pot with 2 tablespoons of oil, then stir in vegetables.

Quick spaghetti with zucchini and hazelnut

Vegetables and pasta make a great combination, especially when hazelnuts and pesto are added to the mix.

Ingredients (4 servings)

Spaghetti for four
3 tbsp olive oil
1 large red or white onion, chopped
4 small zucchinis, unpeeled and diced
Salt and pepper to taste
½ cup hazelnuts, toasted and coarsely chopped
4 tbsp pesto
4 tbsp plain yogurt

A little something extra

▌ Add mushrooms to the zucchini mix.

Preparation

▌ Cook pasta in salted boiling water until *al dente*.

▌ Meanwhile, in a frying pan, heat oil and sauté onion. Cover and cook 5 minutes on low heat.

▌ Add zucchini and cook covered 5 more minutes. Add salt and pepper.

▌ Incorporate hazelnuts, pesto and yogurt. If sauce is too thick, add a bit of cooking water from pasta.

▌ Once the pasta is cooked, drain and return to pot. Pour in sauce and mix well.

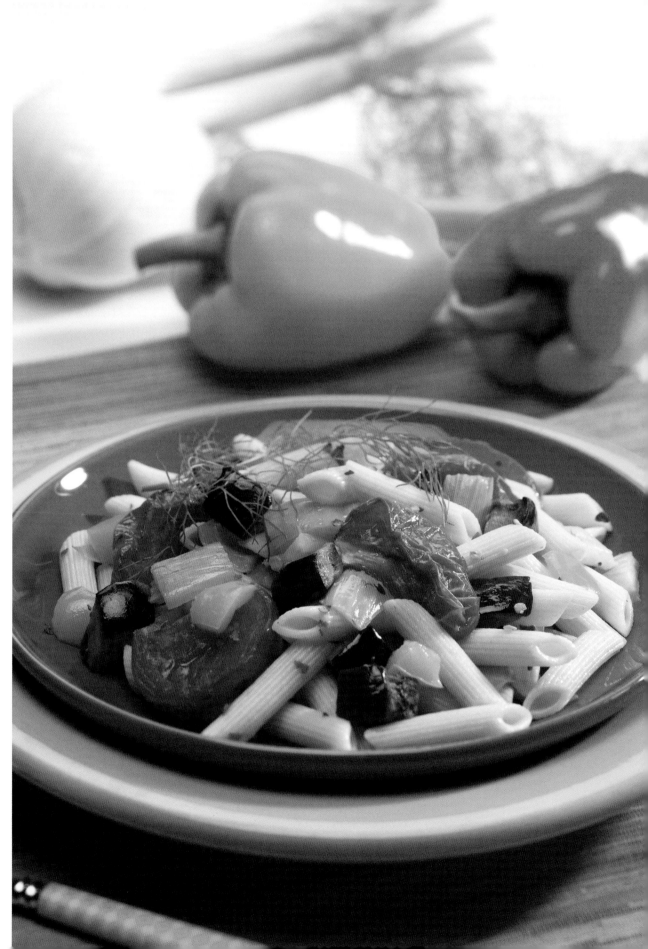

Pasta with sweet pepper coulis

Cooking sweet peppers in the microwave makes them easier to digest and brings out their full flavor.

Ingredients (4 servings)

3 sweet red peppers, cut in three, seeded, white membrane removed
1 clove of garlic, minced
½ cup chicken broth (p. 145)
⅓ cup parmesan
2 tbsp olive oil
2 tbsp yogurt
¼ tsp chili flakes
Fresh basil leaves, chopped
1 tsp dried oregano
1 tsp dried thyme
Salt and pepper to taste
4 tbsp fresh parsley, chopped
¼ cup pecans, chopped (optional)
1 lb pasta of choice

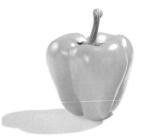

Preparation

■ In a microwave-safe dish (like a Pyrex pie plate), place sweet pepper pieces cut side down. Cover loosely with plastic wrap and microwave on high 12 to 15 minutes until tender but not blackened. Wait 10 minutes before peeling the flesh out with a knife. Repeat until all sweet pepper pieces are cooked.

■ In food processor or mixer, combine garlic, peeled sweet pepper, chicken broth, half of the parmesan, olive oil, yogurt, chili flakes and herbs; purée.

■ Pour the coulis in a small saucepan and heat on the stovetop, or in the microwave in a 4-cup container. Season to taste, add the remaining parmesan and the parsley.

■ In a pot of boiling salted water, cook pasta according to cooking time indicated on package until *al dente*.

■ Drain and incorporate sweet pepper coulis. Garnish with toasted pecans if desired (5 to 10 minutes in a 350°F oven) and serve immediately.

Sweet peppers

Very high in vitamin C and beta-carotein, the sweet pepper also contains mineral salts and vitamin B complex. The combination of vitamin C and beta-carotein helps prevent cataracts, making sweet peppers an ideal choice for aging foodies.

Lasagna roll-ups with pistachios and artichoke hearts

Pasta lovers are sure to fall for this fun variation, filled with a blend of ricotta, artichokes and pistachios.

Ingredients (4 servings)

8 lasagna sheets

Artichoke filling
1 egg, beaten
1 cup low-fat ricotta
4 artichoke hearts, chopped
½ cup pistachios, coarsely chopped
1 tsp lemon zest, grated
¼ tsp nutmeg
Salt and pepper to taste
2 cups tomato sauce (p. 250)
¼ cup gruyère, grated

Preparation

▌ Preheat oven to 375°F.
▌ In a large pot of boiling salted water, cook lasagna until al dente following cooking time on package. Rinse and drain.
▌ In a bowl, combine egg, ricotta, artichoke hearts, pistachios, lemon zest and nutmeg. Season to taste.
▌ Once the lasagna sheets are cooked and drained, cut them in two and put one tablespoon of artichoke mixture on each half. Roll and line them up seam-side down in a rectangular oiled baking dish.
▌ Pour tomato sauce on them and cover with parchment paper.
▌ Bake 20 minutes. Uncover, sprinkle with gruyère and bake another 15 minutes or so until cheese melts to form a golden crust.

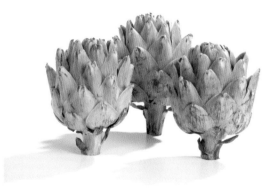

☼ Artichokes

Artichokes are low in fat and rich in fiber. They also contain folic acid, an important nutrient in bone formation and maintenance, as well as magnesium and potassium, two minerals that play an important role in the treatment of arthritis.

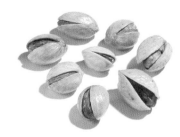

Meatless meat pie in olive oil crust

You will love this tasty vegetarian variation on the French-Canadian tourtière *made with millet, mushrooms, and hazelnuts, and baked in an easy to make pie crust.*

Ingredients (6 servings)

2 tbsp olive oil
1 onion, finely chopped
2 cloves of garlic, minced
2 cups mushrooms, chopped
2 cups cooked millet*
2 tbsp tamari sauce
1 tsp fresh sage, chopped
1 tsp fresh savory, chopped
½ tsp spice mix (coriander, mint, fennel seeds, cayenne pepper)
½ cup hazelnuts, chopped
Salt and pepper to taste

Preparation

▌ In a frying pan, heat oil and lightly brown onion. Add garlic, mushroom, cooked millet, tamari sauce, sage, savory, spice mix, hazelnuts, salt and pepper. If the mixture is too dry, add 1 tbsp of oil and a bit of broth to moisten. Set aside while preparing pie dough.

* *Millet cooks in 15 to 20 minutes: 1 part millet for a little over two parts water.*

Olive oil pie dough

Ingredients (1 double-crust pie)

1 ¾ cups pastry flour, plus an extra ¼ cup
1 ½ tsp salt
1 ½ tsp baking powder
½ cup less 1 tbsp olive oil
½ cup less 1 tbsp unsweetened soy milk
1 large egg, beaten but save ½ tsp of yolk to mix with ½ tsp cold water for egg wash

Preparation

▌ Preheat oven to 425°F.
▌ In a bowl, sift together flour, salt and baking powder. In another bowl, whisk together oil, soy milk and beaten egg.

▌ Pour on dry ingredients and mix with fingers until liquid is absorbed and dough is smooth. Put dough ball in a bowl, cover with plastic wrap and refrigerate at least 30 minutes and up to 3 days.
▌ The dough will be sticky. Knead it mixing in the oil that will have gathered at the bottom of the bowl, add extra flour until easy to handle. Divide in two. Roll out bottom crust on a floured surface to form a circle that will fill a 9-inch pie plate. Fill with millet mixture and drape with rolled out top crust. Brush with egg wash and cut several vents in the top to let steam out.
▌ Bake on bottom grill for 20 minutes, then lower the heat to 375°F and bake 10 minutes more.

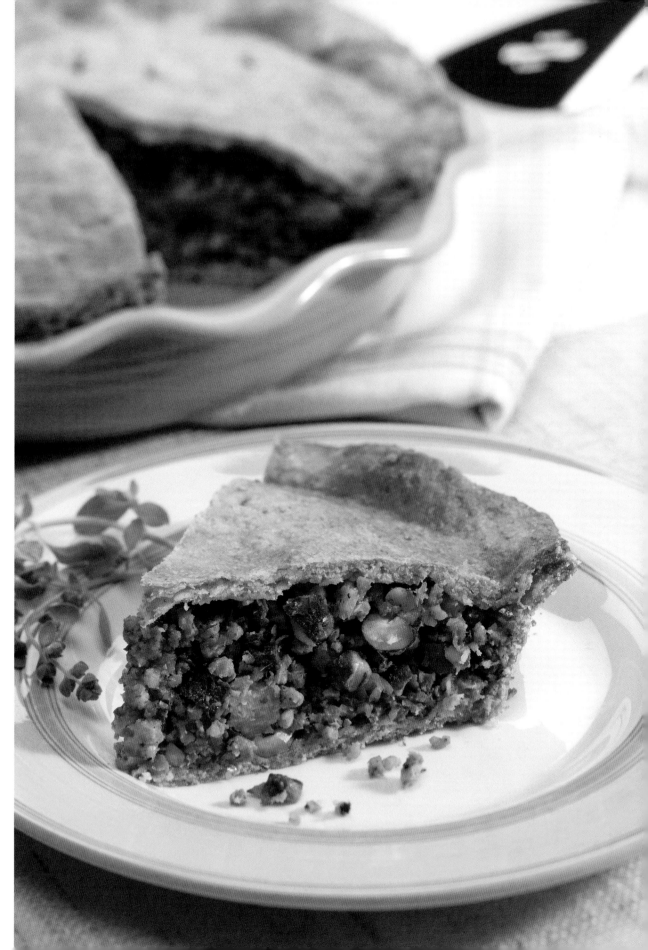

Chickpea and vegetable curry

Go ahead and use any vegetables you might have hiding in the fridge for this spicy curry, such as celery, broccoli, cauliflower, or rutabaga. It will be even tastier if you add dried fruit, or pieces of apple or pineapple.

Ingredients (4 servings)

2 tbsp olive oil
1 large red onion, chopped, or 1 leek (whites), chopped
3 cloves of garlic, minced
2 tbsp fresh ginger, grated
1 tsp curry powder
¼ tsp ground cinnamon
½ tsp turmeric
½ tsp fenugreek (optional)
½ tsp chili flakes
1 tsp lemon zest, grated
19 ounce can chickpeas, rinsed and drained
2 cups chicken broth (p. 145)
2 tbsp tomato paste
1 whole clove (optional)
2 carrots, diced
1 parsnip, diced
1 sweet red pepper and 1 sweet yellow pepper, seeded and diced
2 zucchinis, unpeeled and cubed
½ cup unsalted pistachios, coarsely chopped
2 tbsp cilantro, chopped

Chicken variation

▌ Cut chickpeas by half and replace pistachios with 1 ½ cups of cooked, diced chicken added 5 minutes before done.

Preparation

▌ In a large saucepan, cook onion and leek in oil until golden.

▌ Add garlic, ginger, curry powder, cinnamon, turmeric, fenugreek, chili flakes and lemon zest and sauté for one minute. Add chickpeas, broth, tomato paste, whole clove, carrot, parsnip and sweet pepper.

▌ Cover, bring to a boil, lower heat and simmer 20 minutes. Add zucchini and cook 10 more minutes.

▌ Garnish with pistachios and cilantro. Serve with oven-toasted golden pitas (p. 193).

Tip

▌ Leftovers? Add any leftover curry to a soup for extra flavor.

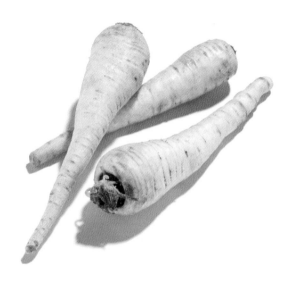

Lentil moussaka

This traditional Greek dish is usually made with ground lamb, but this vegetarian version is just as rich and creamy thanks to the eggplant and the egg sauce.

Ingredients (4 servings)

1 eggplant, sliced
3 tbsp olive oil
1 onion, chopped
1 clove of garlic, minced
19 ounce can lentils, rinsed and drained
8 ounces mushrooms, thinly sliced
2 tbsp tomato paste
28 ounce can diced tomatoes
½ tsp coriander
½ tsp cumin
½ tsp fennel seeds, ground
¼ tsp chili flakes
Salt and pepper to taste
3 tbsp non-hydrogenated margarine
3 tbsp whole wheat flour
1 ½ tasse cups plain unsweetened soy milk
½ tsp each of nutmeg, salt, and pepper
2 eggs, beaten
½ cup gruyère, grated

Preparation

- Preheat oven to 325°F.
- Sprinkle eggplant slices with salt and let sit in a strainer for 30 minutes or so.
- Meanwhile, prepare tomato lentil sauce. Cook onion lightly in oil until translucent but not colored. Add garlic, lentils, mushroom, tomato paste, tomatoes, spices and chili flakes; bring to a boil. Lower heat and cook 30 minutes partially uncovered. Salt only when done.
- While the tomato sauce is cooking, prepare the béchamel. In a small saucepan, melt margarine. Add flour, blend well, then add soy milk and nutmeg. Cook over low heat until mixture thickens. Add salt and pepper.
- Put a bit of this mixture into beaten eggs, one spoonful at a time, to warm eggs gradually, then pour into béchamel and mix well.
- In a baking dish, place the eggplant slices (after wiping the salt off). Add tomato lentil sauce and cover with béchamel. Sprinkle with grated cheese and bake 45 minutes until top is golden.
- Serve with a salad.

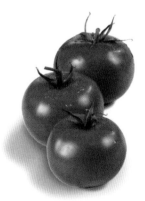

Tomatoes

Contrary to popular belief and despite its acidic taste, the tomato is an alcaline food, which makes it a welcome part in the diet of people suffering from arthritis and gout.

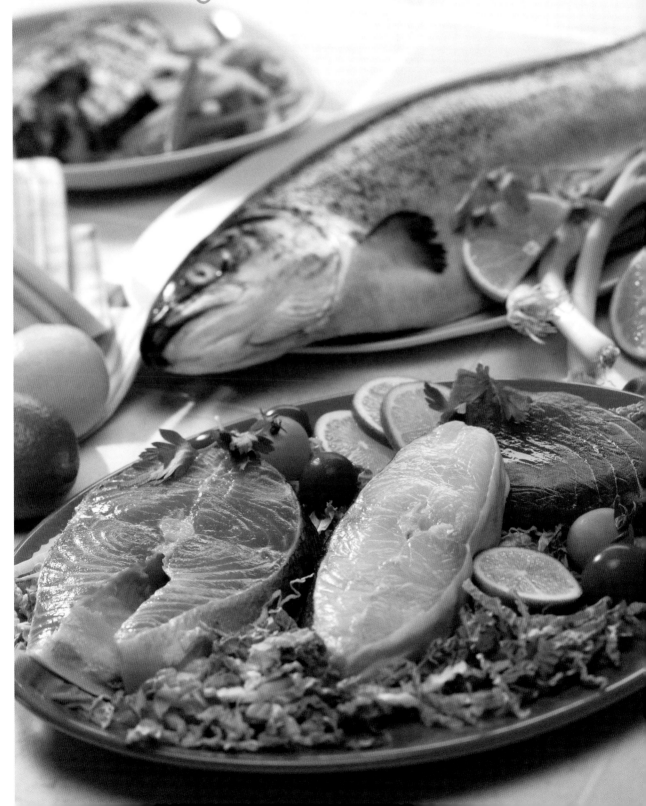

Cooking with fish

From ocean to plate: healthy eating

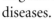e are well aware–but it's still worth mentioning–that countries where fish is a staple food have lower incidences of cardiovascular disease. For this reason only, fish should feature prominently for people trying to maintain a healthy balanced diet. Fortunately for arthritis sufferers, recent research shows that fish is even more beneficial for us because of the omega-3 fatty acids and vitamin B complex it contains–especially oily species like herring, salmon, tuna and sardines. These nutrients are believed to lend anti-inflammatory properties to oily fish making them instrumental in halting the onset of rheumatic diseases.

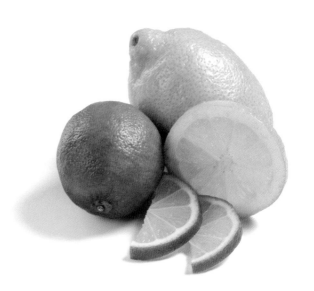

Fish recipes

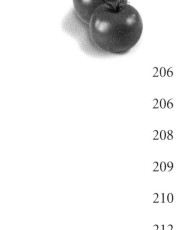

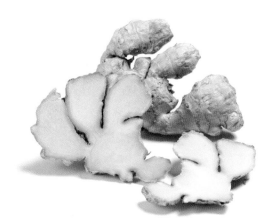

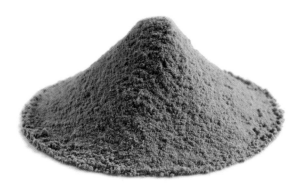

Grilled salmon steaks

Whether cooked on the grill or in the oven, these will satisfy any carnivore's appetite.

Ingredients (4 servings)

4 salmon steaks, 1 inch thick
1 tsp sesame oil
2 tbsp fresh orange juice
1 tbsp tamari sauce
2 tbsp canola oil
4 to 6 tbsp sesame seeds
2 tbsp cilantro leaves, minced

Orange marinade

1 tbsp honey
1 tsp orange marmalade
1 tsp tamari sauce
1 tsp Dijon mustard
2 tbsp walnut oil

Preparation

▌ Combine sesame oil, orange juice, tamari sauce and canola oil. Marinate salmon in mixture for 15 minutes.

▌ Remove salmon from marinade and coat in sesame seeds.

▌ Grill 3 to 5 minutes per side on an electric barbecue (these are healthier than gas grills) or broil in the oven 6 inches from the grill.

Gingered salmon fillets
Cooked in the microwave

Salmon is wonderfully versatile. Cooked in the microwave in an Asian-inspired marinade, it is moist and tender as long as you are careful not to overcook it.

Ingredients (2 servings)

1 tbsp canola oil
4 green onions, chopped
1 tsp sesame oil
1 tbsp tamari sauce
1 tbsp fresh ginger, minced
1 tsp honey
2 tbsp orange juice (or clementine juice)
2 salmon fillets
Pepper to taste

Preparation

▌ In a microwave-safe dish, combine canola oil and green onions. Microwave on high for 1 minute.

▌ Add sesame oil, tamari sauce, ginger, honey, orange juice and mix well before adding salmon. Cover loosely with wax paper.

▌ Microwave on medium-high for 2 minutes. Turn fillets over and cook 1 more minute. Check doneness and continue cooking if necessary.

▌ Let rest 3 minutes before serving.

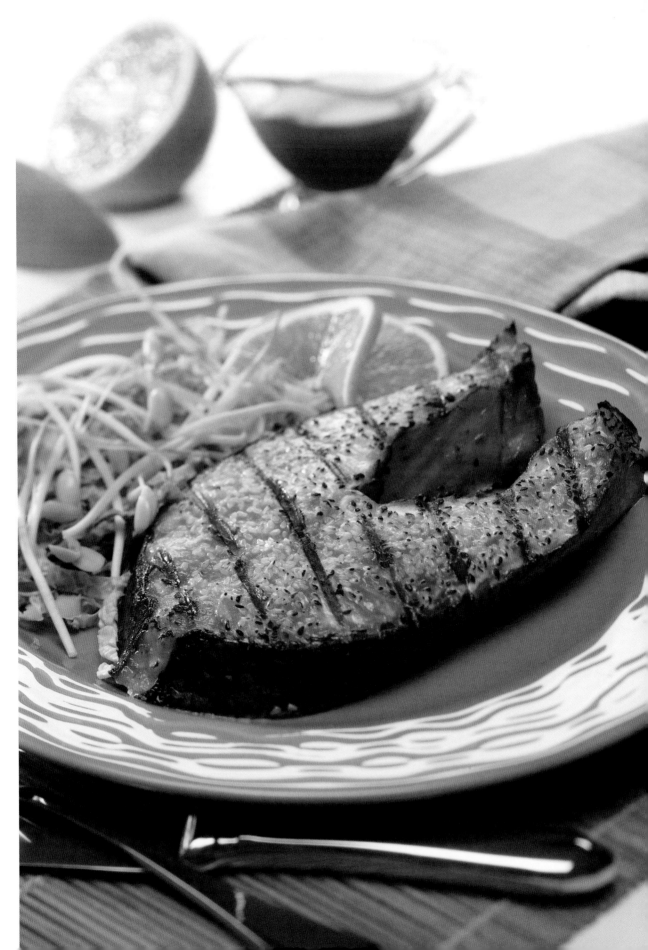

Salmon fillets en chemise

Cooking fish wrapped in a shirt of parchment paper (chemise means "shirt" in French) gives delicate flavors to the meat. This version blends the aromas of tarragon, capers and lemon.

Ingredients (4 servings)

4 salmon fillets

Caper and lemon marinade

3 tbsp olive oil
2 tbsp fresh tarragon
2 tbsp fresh parsley, minced
2 tbsp capers, rinsed, drained and chopped
2 tbsp anchovies, rinsed, drained and chopped
2 tbsp lemon juice
1 tsp lemon zest, grated
Salt and pepper to taste

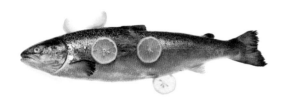

Preparation

- Preheat oven to 400°F.
- In a salad bowl or deep dish, combine all marinade ingredients and mix well. Dip fillets in marinade to coat.
- Place fillets on parchment paper and drizzle with remaining marinade. Fold paper over to wrap fillets into four packets.
- Cook 15 to 20 minutes.

✱ Parchment paper

Used for oven-baking, parchment paper has two advantages over foil: foods won't stick to it and it is non-toxic. It lends itself perfectly to cooking foods in packets, or as the French say "en chemise".

✱ Salmon

Salmon is rich in omega-3 fatty acids and is known for its anti-inflammatory properties. It is also rich in vitamin D, an essential nutrient for bone health.

Barbecue variation

- This marinade is perfect for grilling fish on an electric barbecue. Marinate fillets for 1 hour , then cook 3 minutes per side.

Trout fillets with almond tartar sauce
Cooked in the microwave

Microwave cooking is perfect for fish, leaving it tender and moist. These fillets will be just as delicious with a tomato sauce or an Asian vinaigrette.

Ingredients (2 servings)

2 trout fillets
1 tbsp olive oil
1 tbsp lemon juice
½ tsp tarragon

Almond tartar sauce
¼ cup plain firm yogurt
1 tbsp lemon juice
1 tsp lemon zest, grated
2 tbsp capers
2 tbsp dill pickles, chopped
2 tbsp almonds, ground
½ tsp fennel seeds, ground
Salt and pepper to taste

Preparation

▌ In a microwave-safe dish, combine oil, lemon juice and fillets. Cover with wax paper and microwave on medium-high for 3 minutes, turning over half way.

▌ Meanwhile, combine tartar sauce ingredients in a small bowl. Taste and adjust seasoning. Serve with fish fillets and a green vegetable or salad of your choice.

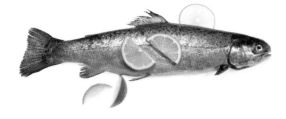

Firm yogurt

▌ If you want firm yogurt with cheese-like consistency, wrap it in a cheesecloth or muslin-lined strainer and put it in the fridge for 6 hours to drain the water out.

Trout

Researchers have concluded that wild trout is a better source of omega-3 fatty acids than farmed trout due to the differences in the fishes' diets.

Trout fillets with green peppercorns and curry sauce
Cooked in the microwave

Served with a fragrant and tasty sauce, these fillets melt in your mouth. Delicious on white rice accompanied by green beans.

Ingredients (4 servings)

1 tbsp non-hydrogenated margarine
1 tbsp peppercorns, packed in vinegar
2 tbsp lime juice
4 trout fillets

Curry sauce

2 tbsp non-hydrogenated margarine
1 dry shallot, minced
2 tbsp flour
½ tsp turmeric
1 tsp curry powder
¼ tsp curry paste
1 cup chicken broth (p. 145)
4 tbsp fresh parsley, chopped
Salt and pepper to taste

Preparation

▌ Start by preparing the curry sauce. In a small saucepan, melt 2 tbsp of margarine and gently sauté onion. Sprinkle in flour, turmeric and blend in curry powder and curry paste. Cook 1 or 2 minutes. Pour in chicken broth and cook while stirring until mixture thickens.

▌ In a microwave-safe Pyrex pie plate, melt the other tablespoon of margarine for 45 seconds. Add lemon juice and peppercorns, then put fillets in. Loosely cover with plastic wrap and microwave at medium-high for 3 minutes. Turn fillets over and cook for another minute or two. Check doneness and continue cooking if needed, 1 minute at a time.

▌ Let rest 2 minutes before serving fillets draped with curry sauce.

Variation

▌ Fish of all kinds can be cooked this way and served with an infinite choice of sauces and garnishes, tartar, tomatoes, pesto, herbs, etc.

✷ Curry paste

Curry paste is available in both yellow and red varieties and is sold in most supermarkets in the exotic food aisle.

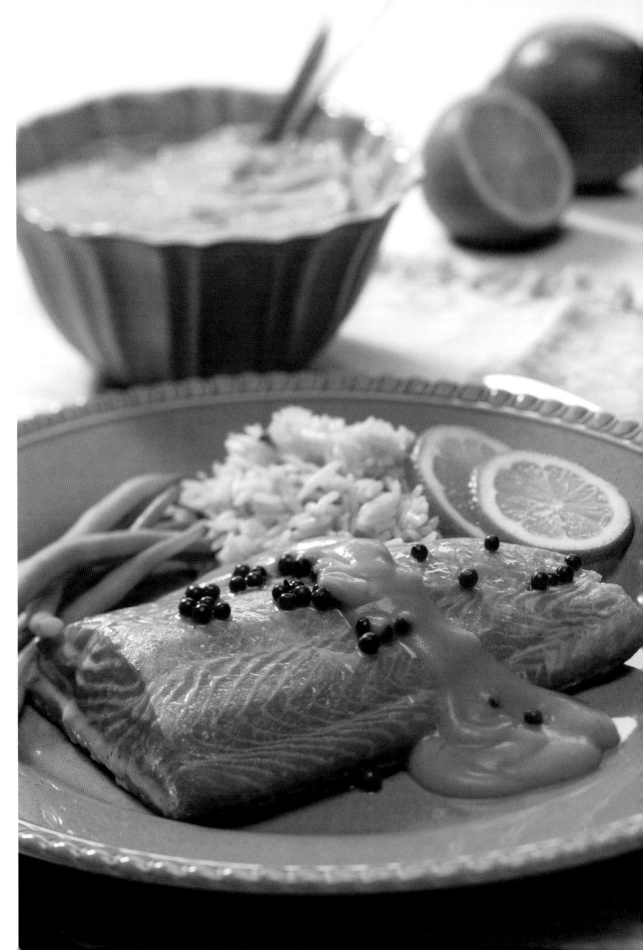

Sardine linguine

Pasta and sardines , a truly unusual combination that is surprisingly delicious.

Ingredients (4 servings)

2 tbsp olive oil

8 ounces mushrooms, chopped finely

2-ounce can anchovy fillets, rinsed, drained and chopped

2 cups tomato sauce (p. 250)

2 cans (4.5 ounces each) sardines packed in olive oil, drained and chopped

¼ cup fresh parsley, chopped

¾ lb linguine

Salt and pepper to taste

Preparation

▌ In a small saucepan, heat oil and sauté mushrooms. Add anchovies and tomato sauce. Bring to a boil, lower heat and simmer 10 minutes, uncovered.

▌ Meanwhile, cook pasta *al dente* following instructions as indicated on package.

▌ When sauce is done simmering, add sardines and parsley, season to taste and heat for 5 minutes.

▌ Serve sardine sauce on drained pasta.

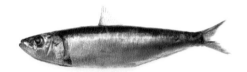

❀ Canned sardines

It is recommended to add sardines to a balanced diet even though many of them are imported. Most canned sardines are actually small herring. Either way, they are full of omega-3s , almost as much as fresh sardines.

❀ Anchovies

Anchovies are small, oily fish that are high in calories. They feature prominently in Mediterranean cuisines to enhance the flavors of tapenade, soups, fish dishes, pasta dishes and more.

Poached turbot with fresh tomatoes

Poached on a bed of fresh vegetables, this fish is quick and easy to make, and oh so good.

Ingredients (4 servings)

4 turbot steaks
Salt and pepper to taste
2 tbsp olive oil
1 red or white onion, finely chopped
2 cloves of garlic, minced
4 tomatoes, peeled, seeded and chopped
2 tbsp fresh basil, chopped
2 tbsp fresh parsley, chopped
½ cup dry white wine

Preparation

▌ Season the fish with salt and pepper.
▌ In a frying pan, heat oil and lightly brown onion over low heat, stirring occasionally.
▌ Add garlic and tomatoes, then season. Increase heat and cook for 5 minutes.
▌ Put fish on top of tomatoes and pour wine over them.
▌ Cover and bring to a boil over medium heat. As soon as it begins to boil, lower heat and turn fish over. Cover and simmer 3 to 5 minutes.
▌ Put fish on a serving platter and keep warm.
▌ Add basil and parsley, boil the remaining liquid over high heat to thicken sauce. Pour sauce over fish and serve immediately.

Gourmet touch

▌ Add 4 tablespoons of diced feta cheese when adding the herbs.

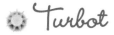

Turbot

Turbot's delicate white meat is greatly appreciated by gourmets. It is also rich in omega-3 fatty acids, nutrients that give the fish its anti-inflammatory properties.

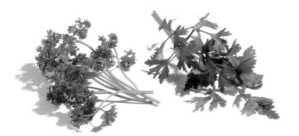

Parsley

An aromatic plant that is most often used as a garnish, has many therapeutic properties and is very useful in promoting joint health and flexibility. With its high concentration of vitamins A, B, C, and calcium, it is a perfect food for arthritis sufferers.

Grilled bluefin tuna marinated in soy and ginger

To fully appreciate tuna, the filet mignon of fish, it is best eaten almost raw as it is in Asia. The easiest way to cook it just right is in the oven for a few minutes then finishing it off on the grill.

Ingredients (4 servings)

1 tbsp olive oil
4 thick slices of bluefin tuna
6 tbsp (or so) sesame seeds, toasted

Ginger marinade

2 tbsp fresh ginger, minced
4 green onions, chopped
2 tbsp cilantro, chopped
2 cloves of garlic, minced
2 tbsp tamari sauce
4 tbsp canola oil
2 tbsp sesame oil
Salt and pepper to taste (be careful , tamari sauce is very salty)

Preparation

- Preheat oven to 425°F.
- Make marinade by mixing all the ingredients in a deep plate, big enough for the fish.
- Put the fish in the marinade and let sit for 1 hour at room temperature.
- In a small plate, pour sesame seeds. Remove fish from marinade and press in the seeds to coat both sides.
- In an oven-safe frying pan, heat oil and cook fish for 1 minute on each side. Put pan in the oven and cook 3 to 5 minutes depending on the thickness, making sure not to overcook. Serve with the vegetable packets (p. 237) you will have cooked in the oven before the fish.

Sesame oil

This nutty tasting oil contains a good balance of oleic acid and omega-6s. It also contains sesamin and sesamolin which give the oil its antioxidant properties.

Tuna

It would be quite difficult to confuse albacore tuna–the kind that comes in cans–and bluefin tuna, an oily fish that is available fresh between July and September, to the delight of foodies everywhere. The bluefin has superior meat and arthritis sufferers will benefit from this omega-3 rich fish.

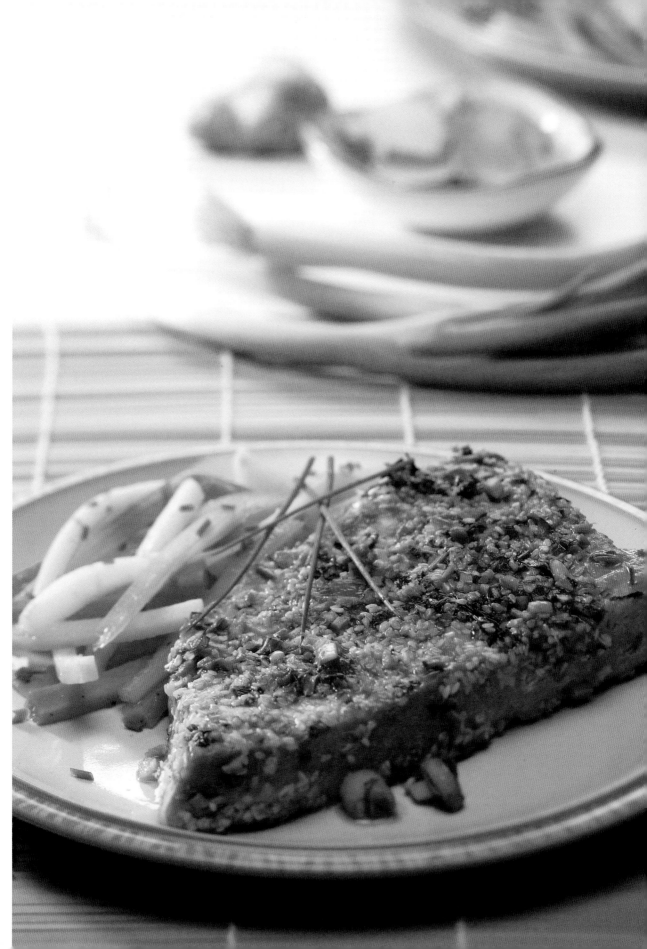

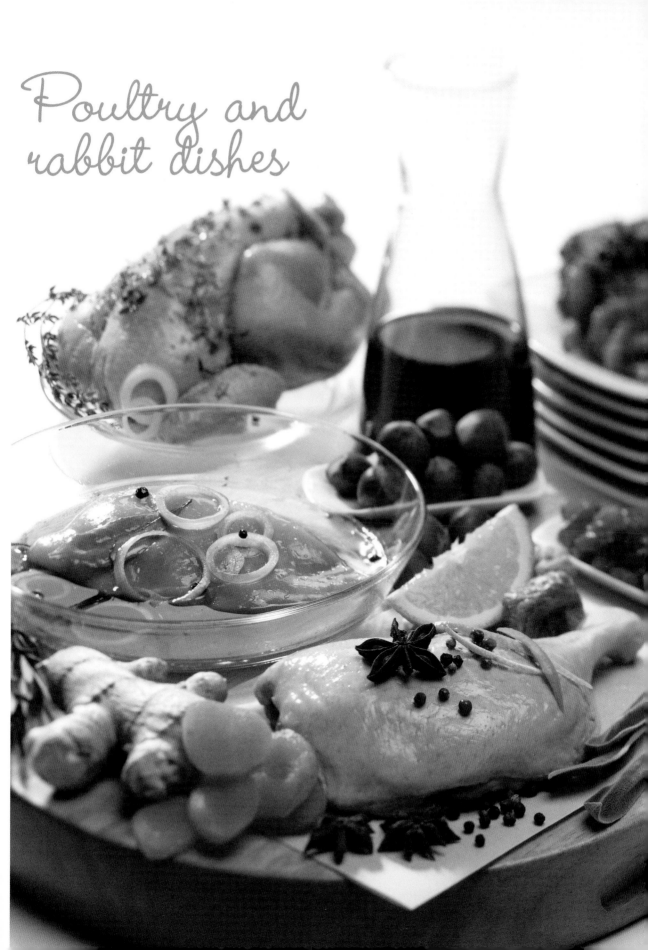

Poultry and
rabbit dishes

Indulgent dishes

$\mathcal{M}$eat is not very good for arthritis sufferers, particularly processed and red meats because of their high saturated fat content that can contribute to aggravating inflammation. But this is not the case for poultry and rabbit, which haven't yet shown any undesirable side effects in people with different forms of rheumatic disorders. A multitude of poultry recipes exist. I chose the ones I thought would be good to serve to impress guests without compromising your new joint-friendly diet.

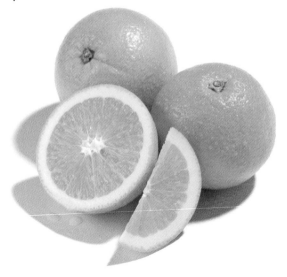

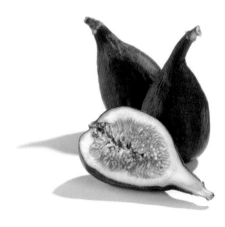

Poultry and rabbit dishes

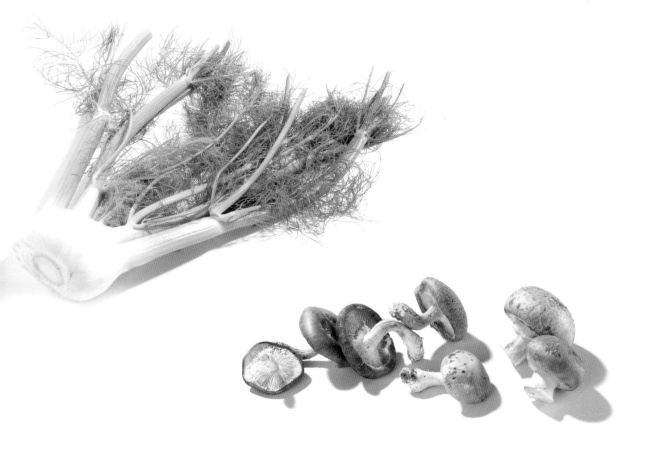

Layered chicken and eggplant

This dish is easier than it looks, and will satisfy the most discriminating palate.

Ingredients for 4

2 eggs
1 tbsp water
⅔ cup seasoned bread crumbs
3 tbsp fresh parsley, finely chopped
1 tbsp parmesan, grated
1 large eggplant, cut in four lenghtwise
2 large chicken breasts, cut lenghtwise in cutlets
2 tbsp olive oil
½ cup tomato sauce (p. 250)
½ cup gruyère, grated

Preparation

▌ Preheat oven to 425°F.

▌ In a deep plate, beat eggs with water. In another deep plate, combine bread crumbs, parsley and parmesan. Dip eggplant slices in egg, then dredge in bread crumbs.

▌ Put eggplant slices on an oiled baking sheet and cook 20 minutes, turning over halfway through. (This is a very tasty way to cook eggplant; if you want to make this a vegetarian dish, just omit the chicken.)

▌ Meanwhile, dip chicken cutlets in egg, then dredge in bread crumbs. Heat oil and cook chicken cutlets about 5 minutes, turning over halfway through.

▌ Put a tablespoon of tomato sauce on each eggplant slice, then add a piece of chicken and top with another tablespoon of sauce.

▌ Sprinkle with grated cheese and repeat the process with the rest of the eggplant and chicken slices. Cook in the oven for 5 minutes or until cheese is melted.

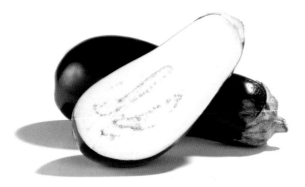

✳ Eggplant

This beautiful and richly-colored vegetable is easy to digest and low in calories. According to nutrition experts, eating eggplant after a meal full of fats can help prevent lipids and cholesterol levels in the blood from rising.

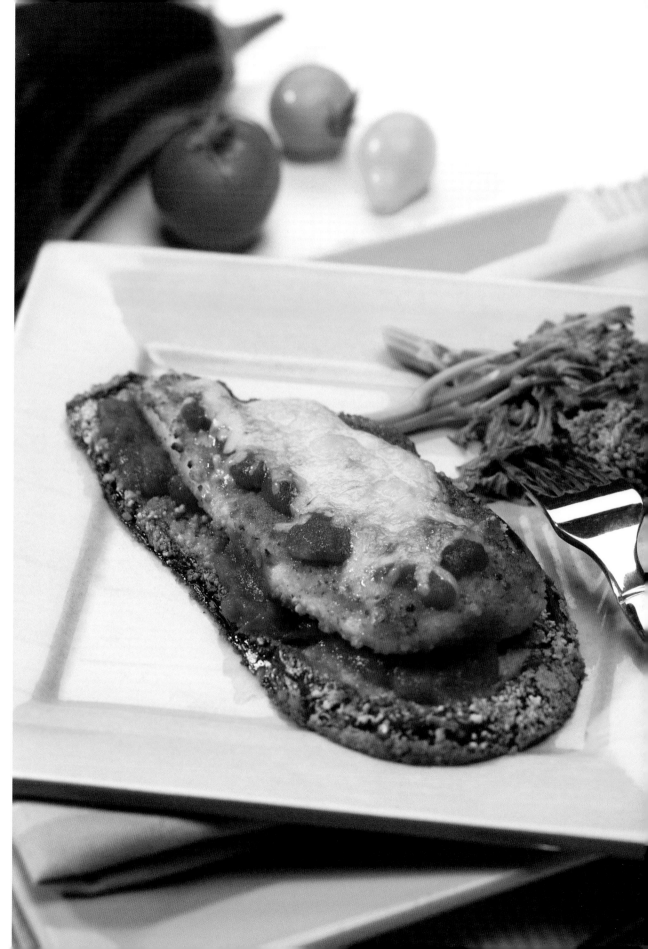

Roast chicken

The most simple recipes are often the ones that keep us coming back for more. I have been going back to this recipe for years and it is still as delicious.

Ingredients (4 servings)

1 grain-fed, air-chilled chicken (approx. 2 lbs)
Half a lemon
1 carrot, cut in pieces
1 small onion, halved
1 clove of garlic
2 tbsp olive oil
1 tsp mixed herbs (oregano, thyme, paprika)
¼ cup white wine

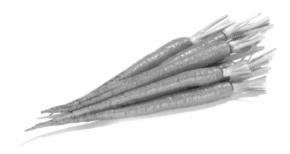

Chicken

Chicken meat is deliciously light and pleasing, and when eaten without the skin, it is low in calories. It is a good source of protein and vitamin B complex. Chicken bones contain collagen which is known to alleviate rheumatoid arthritis symptoms.

Preparation

- Preheat the oven to 350°F.
- Rub chicken with the lemon half and dry off. Put the carrot, onion and garlic inside the chicken, add half of the herb mix with salt and pepper. Cross the legs and tie them together with wire.
- Put chicken in a baking pan, brush with olive oil and rest of herbs.
- Cook 1 ½ hours, drizzling with 1 or 2 tablespoons of white wine every 30 minutes.
- Serve with mashed parsnip, carrot, and sweet potato (p. 240).

Gourmet variation

- Surround chicken with fennel bulbs sliced in four that have been boiled for 10 minutes in salt water.

Tip

- Don't waste any part of this flavorful dish; use leftover sauce and carcass to make broth (p. 145).

Hurray for leftovers!

- Try the *Tortilla cup with curried chicken* recipe on page 179.

Duck en chemise with salted herbs

As tender as duck confit, this dish is a pure delight that will tantalize the gourmet palate.

Ingredients (4 servings)

1 duck, cut in 6 pieces
2 tbsp olive oil
3 cloves of garlic, minced
2 tbsp olive oil
3 tsp salted herbs
Dash of ground cloves
Zest of 1 orange, grated
2 cups coarse salt
Parchment paper and foil

Waste not, want not

- Make broth with the leftover carcass (p. 145).
- Make pâté with the duck liver that you put aside (p. 228).

Salted herbs

Made with a mix of fresh herbs (chives, savory, parsley, thyme and celery leaves), salted herbs lend their summer flavors to soups, stews and sauces. Moreover, commercially-packed salted herbs only contain salt as a preservative.

Preparation

- Preheat oven to 450°F.
- In a large frying pan, heat oil over medium heat and cook duck pieces 5 minutes or until golden brown. While the duck is cooking, prick skin with a knife or skewer.
- In a small bowl, mix garlic, 2 tbsp of olive oil, salted herbs, clove and orange zest.
- When duck is cooked, place each piece on a square of parchment paper twice its size.
- Top duck pieces with salted herbs and fold paper over to make packets. Wrap parchment paper packets in foil carefully to prevent juices from running out.
- In a baking pan large enough to contain all the packets, pour in salt and lay packets down on top.
- Cook for 1 hour. Serve with baked potatoes.

Duck thighs with dried fruit

Cooked in a fragrant infusion of orange and spices, these duck thighs are not only delicious, but also easy to make.

Ingredients (2 servings)

1 cup of freshly-brewed green tea
10 dried apricots
2 dried figs
4 peppercorns
1 star anise
1 whole clove
1 knob of ginger, peeled and thinly slices
   (about 2 tbsp)
Zest of 1 orange, cut in thin strips
1 tbsp olive oil
2 duck thighs
½ tsp spice mix (mint, coriander, cardamom)
Salt and pepper to taste

Preparation

▌ In hot tea, add apricots, figs, peppercorns, star anise, clove, ginger slices and orange zest. Let rest at room temperature for 4 hours or overnight.

▌ In a frying pan, heat oil and cook duck thighs over medium heat until golden brown, about 5 minutes on each side. Add spice mix, salt and pepper.

▌ Meanwhile, remove fruit and ginger from tea and slice fruit thinly. Add to the duck along with a third of the tea, setting orange zest aside.

▌ Cover, bring to a boil, lower heat and simmer duck thighs over low heat for 1 ½ hours. If more liquid is needed, pour in more tea.

▌ Once the duck is tender, transfer to a dish with fruit and keep warm.

▌ Discard cooking liquid, deglaze pan with remaining tea, add orange zest and reduce.

▌ Serve duck thighs and fruit draped with this sauce, accompanied with mashed sweet potatoes or rice.

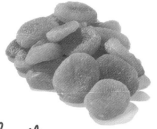

✸ Dried fruit

Dehydrating fruit allows them to retain most of their vitamins and greatly increases their fiber content. The preservation process that removes the water they contain increases their energy value, and also increases their caloric value compared to fresh fruit. They make a great snack for active people who can add them to morning cereal for extra energy. They are a welcomed addition to stews and braised dishes of all kinds by giving them a fragrant aroma and taste.

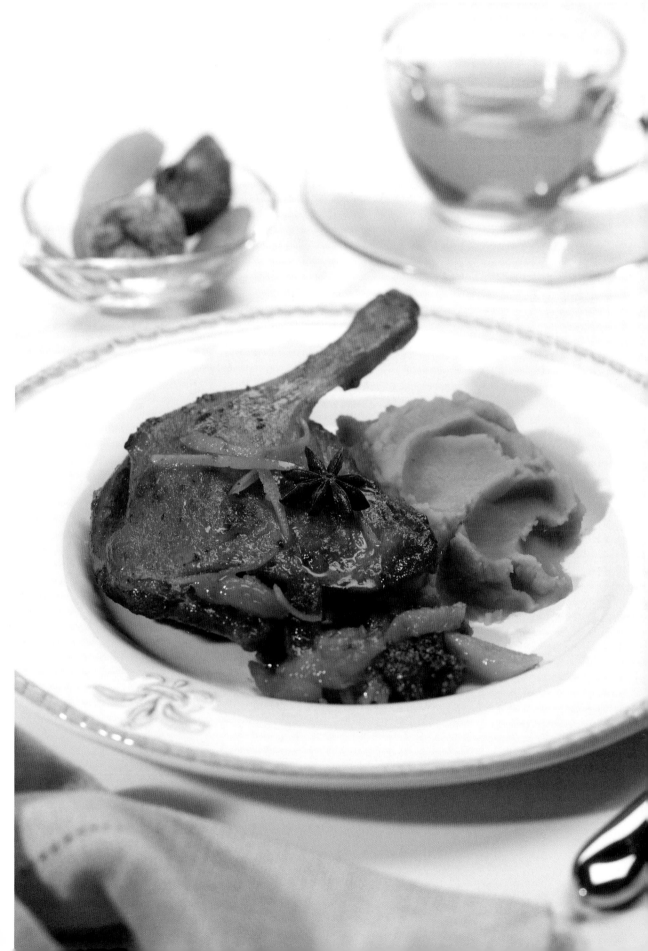

Rabbit with dried fruit

This a classic English dish that I have been making and enjoying for many years, proving that British cooking is not at all flavorless and boring.

Ingredients (4 servings)

1 rabbit (4 lbs) in pieces
4 tbsp olive oil
½ tsp dried thyme
½ tsp dried rosemary
1 tbsp mustard
1 tbsp cornstarch, dissolved in 2 tbsp light
  cream
½ cup port wine
½ cup raisins
½ cup hazelnuts, coarsely chopped
2 tbsp fresh parsley, chopped
Salt and pepper to taste

Marinade
1 cup white wine or apple juice
¼ cup olive oil
10 ounces of prunes
2 cloves of garlic, minced
1 onion, minced
1 carrot, sliced

Preparation

▌ Combine all marinade ingredients in a large shallow dish and mix well. Add the rabbit pieces and marinate for 6 hours at room temperature, turning over once in a while.

▌ Remove rabbit pieces and dry them off with some paper towel. Reserve marinade.

▌ In a large saucepan, heat olive oil and cook rabbit pieces over medium heat until lightly golden (about 10 minutes). Add marinade and bring to a boil; lower heat and simmer one hour over very low heat.

▌ Remove rabbit pieces and keep warm. Strain cooking liquid and return to saucepan. Discard bits and pieces left in the strainer. Incorporate thyme, rosemary, mustard and dissolved cornstarch; stir gently over medium heat. Add port, raisins and hazelnuts and simmer 10 minutes.

▌ Warm rabbit pieces up in the sauce, garnish with fresh parsley and serve with short pasta or with mashed potatoes and a green vegetable.

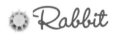 Rabbit

Rabbit meat is low in fat and high in protein, and is very similar to chicken meat, but more tender and tastier. It should be favored by arthritis sufferers for its high content of vitamins and minerals.

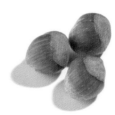

Tarragon rabbit

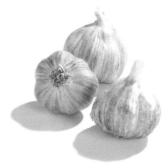

Quite a rich dish due to the combination of cream and white wine, but your joints will suffer less if you serve it after a nice salad of papaya, mango and kiwi (p. 166).

Ingredients (4 servings)

1 rabbit (3 lbs)
3 tbsp flour (or more)
3 tbsp olive oil
3 dry shallots, peeled and quartered
3 cloves of garlic, minced
1 cup white wine
1 cup chicken broth (p. 145)
2 tbsp fresh tarragon (or 2 tsp dried tarragon)
1 tbsp Dijon mustard
1 tsp cornstarch
¼ cup 15% table cream
Salt and pepper to taste

Preparation

- Preheat oven to 350°F.
- Dredge rabbit pieces in flour.
- In a large baking dish, heat oil and gently cook rabbit until golden. Remove from dish and set aside.
- Add shallots and sauté a few minutes, then sauté garlic for 1 minute. Add wine, broth and tarragon; cover, bring to a boil and add rabbit pieces. Season and cook in oven for 1 ½ hours.
- Remove rabbit and shallots, and keep warm.
- Dissolve cornstarch in the cream and add mustard. Warm up cooking juices and moisten with cream and mustard mixture. Heat until thickened.
- Adjust seasoning and drape over rabbit pieces.
- Serve with short pasta sprinkled with parsley accompanied with lemony green beans (p. 236).

Tip

- If the rabbit still has a liver, keep it and use it to make a delicious pâté (p. 228).

Tarragon

This delicately aromatic plant contains iron, manganese, calcium and vitamin C. Tarragon is said to promote digestion, clean the intestinal tract, calm the nervous system, and fight insomnia. It pairs very well with mushrooms and adds fragrant aroma to quiches, chicken, veal, white-fleshed fish and salmon. It is a good salt substitute in a salad.

Rabbit à l'orange with ginger

This delectable dish is easy to make–and easy to eat! If you don't like the taste of ginger,
replace the ginger marmalade with orange marmalade.

Ingredients (4 servings)

1 rabbit (3 lbs) cut in 6 pieces and floured
2 tbsp flour
3 tbsp olive oil and a bit more
2 onions, quartered
1 cup orange juice
½ cup red wine
1 tbsp balsamic vinegar
1 tbsp ginger marmalade
4 small, fresh sage leaves
1 cup chicken broth (p. 145)
Salt and pepper to taste
1 tsp cornstarch

Preparation

▌ Preheat oven to 350°F.

▌ In an oven-proof saucepan, heat oil and cook rabbit pieces. When they are golden brown, transfer to a dish and set aside. Discard cooking juices, add more oil to the saucepan and sauté onions. Add all other ingredients except cornstarch. Add rabbit pieces, season to taste, cover and bring to a boil.

▌ Bake in oven, covered, for 1 ½ hours or until rabbit is tender.

▌ To make the sauce, take 1 cup of liquid from saucepan, strain, dissolve cornstarch into it, and bring gently to a boil. Simmer a few minutes until thickened.

▌ Drape the sauce on rabbit pieces and garnish with sage leaves.

Quick liver pâté

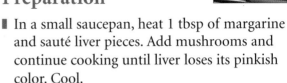

Ingredients (4 servings)

Poultry or rabbit liver, denerved and coarsel chopped
2 tbsp non-hydrogenated margarine and a little extra
¼ cup pistachios, shelled
¼ cup mushrooms, chopped
½ tsp lemon zest, grated
½ tsp Maghrebian spice mix
Salt and pepper to taste

Preparation

▌ In a small saucepan, heat 1 tbsp of margarine and sauté liver pieces. Add mushrooms and continue cooking until liver loses its pinkish color. Cool.

▌ In a small grinder, coarsely grind pistachios. Add cooked liver and mushrooms; grind.

▌ Put mixture in a terrine. Add remaining margarine, lemon zest, spice mix, salt and pepper. If pâté appears too dry, add a bit more margarine.

▌ Mix and refrigerate for 1 hour before serving.

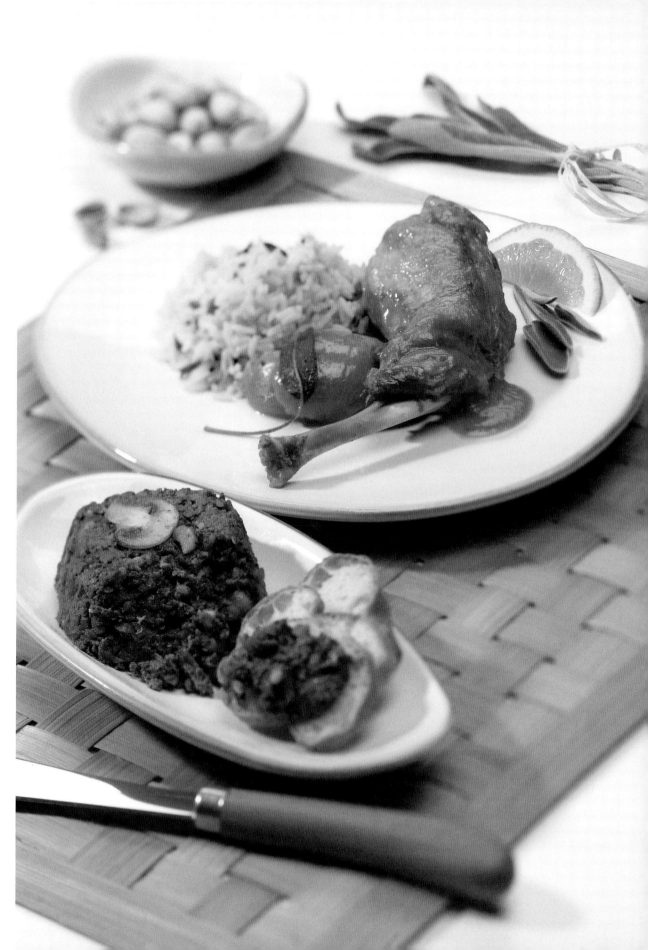

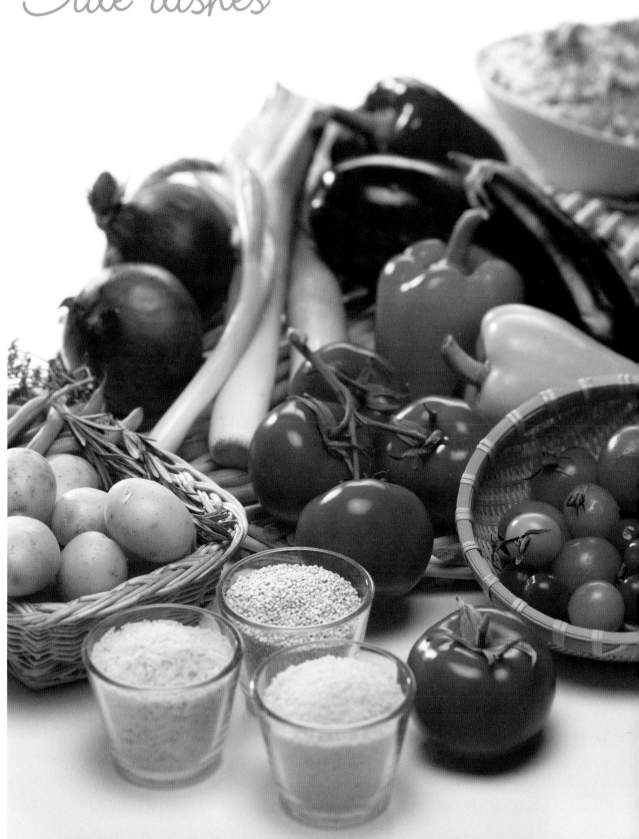

Side dishes

Perfect companions

The perfect companion–or sidekick–to any dish is discreet food, happy in a supporting role. It will not only make the main dish shine, but will also help balance out the meal if it's too rich in fat. Vegetables are ideal in a meal where meat is the star because they can counteract the bad fats contained in many meat dishes thanks to their fiber and antioxidant content. If you eat several meat-based meals in a week, make sure you load up on vegetables. Check out the vegetable section of this book to discover new varieties and include as many as possible on the table. Grains are another healthy ally, especially for those who eat smaller meals or who want to benefit from grains' many therapeutic properties.

Side dishes

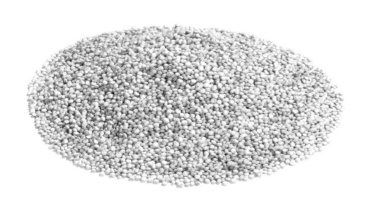

Beets infused with orange
Cooked in the microwave

This quick-to-make side dish is rich in iron and potassium, two nutrients that help maintain healthy bones. It is a delicious dish served with grilled poultry or fish.

Ingredients (4 servings)

2 tbsp olive oil
14 ounce can whole beets, diced
2 tbsp orange or clementine juice
1 tsp orange zest, grated
1 tsp honey
½ tsp turmeric
2 tsp sesame seeds

Preparation

▌ In a microwave-safe bowl, combine beets, juice, zest, honey and turmeric.

▌ Cover with wax paper and microwave on medium-high for 2 minutes.

▌ Divide into 4 small bowls or ramekins, garnish with sesame seeds and serve.

Lemon and nut couscous

Couscous, or precooked wheat semolina, is very versatile and goes really well with fish. Here is a lovely couscous dish infused with fragrant lemon and cilantro.

Ingredients (6 servings)

2 cups couscous
2 ¼ cups boiling water
½ tsp hot sauce
Zest of 1 lemon, grated
½ cup nuts, toasted (pine nuts or pistachios)
½ cup cilantro leaves, chopped

Preparation

▌ Stir couscous in salted boiling water with hot sauce, and let stand 5 minutes. Fluff with a fork. Add nuts, lemon zest and cilantro leaves. Heat 2 to 3 minutes in the microwave and serve with fish, poultry or grilled meat.

☀ Couscous

The small wheat semolina pellet known as couscous is low in fat and salt. It is a good source of plant protein, fiber and vitamin B3. It cooks in 5 minutes and goes just as well with fruit as with vegetables to make light, refreshing salads.

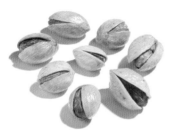

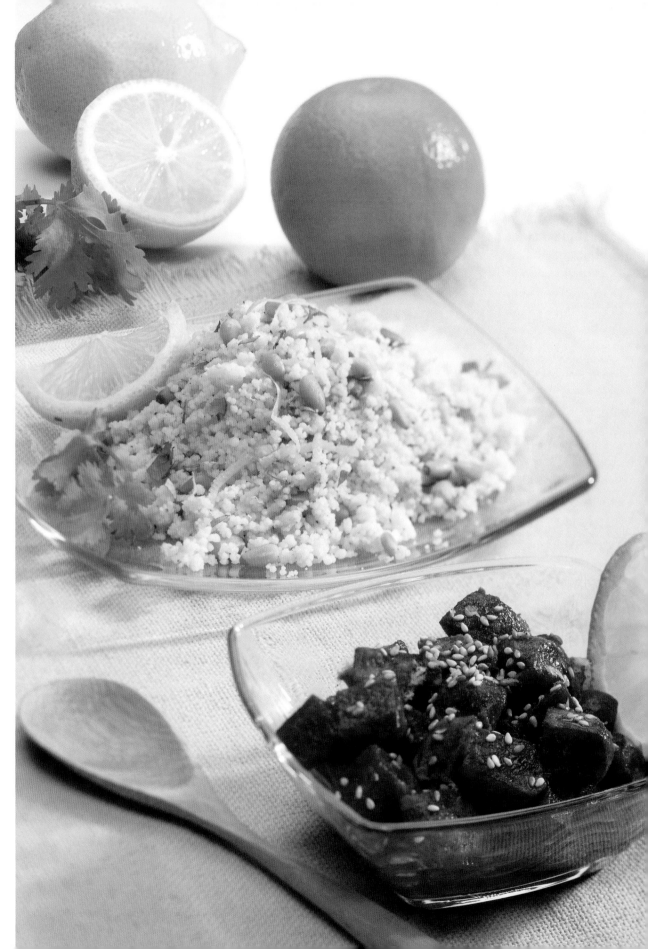

Oven fries

Lovers of fries rejoice! This version calls for a very small quantity of oil so you can still enjoy a favorite treat, but make sure you don't overindulge!

Ingredients (2 servings,
or 3 smaller ones)

3 medium potatoes, peeled and julienned
1 tbsp canola oil
½ tsp paprika
½ tsp chili seasoning
½ tsp salt
¼ tsp pepper

Preparation

▌ Preheat oven to 450°F.
▌ In a salad bowl, combine oil, paprika, chili seasoning, salt and pepper. Add potatoes and mix with your hands.
▌ On a large baking sheet covered in parchment paper, spread potatoes out in a single layer.
▌ Cook 20 minutes in the oven. Check doneness and continue cooking if necessary.

Lemony green beans with almonds

Say goodbye to limp, canned beans and enjoy these aromatic and crunchy delights.

Ingredients (4 servings)

1 lb green beans, trimmed
2 tbsp slivered almonds
¼ cup fresh parsley, chopped
1 tbsp olive oil
1 tbsp lemon juice
1 tsp lemon zest, grated
Salt and pepper to taste

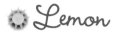 **Lemon**

Lemon juice and rind are widely used in cooking, bringing their flavor to everything from soups to desserts. I use lemon juice liberally in many of my recipes and could not do without the zest. Research has shown that lemon's antioxidant properties may help prevent cancer growth and delay the symptoms of aging.

Preparation

▌ In a steamer or in a pot of boiling salt water, cook beans for 15 minutes.
▌ Meanwhile, toast almonds 5 to 10 minutes in a 350°F oven until golden.
▌ In a small bowl, combine parsley, oil, lemon juice and zest, salt and pepper.
▌ Pour this mixture on *al dente* beans and sprinkle with almonds.
▌ Heat 1 minute in microwave before serving.

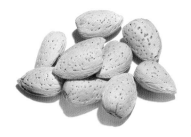

Honeyed root vegetables

This delicious way to eat root vegetable is also very convenient; the vegetables roast alongside the chicken they will accompany at the table.

Ingredients (4 servings)

2 tbsp olive oil
2 tbsp honey
1 tsp Dijon mustard
1 leek (whites), minced
4 cups vegetables, diced or julienned (carrot, parsnip, rutabaga, potato)
1 tbsp mixed dried herbs (thyme, sage, oregano, savory)
Salt and pepper to taste

Preparation

▮ Preheat oven to 350°F.
▮ In a large oven-proof skillet, heat oil, honey and mustard. Sauté leek whites, then add the other vegetables, salt and pepper. Cook over medium heat for 5 minutes.
▮ Transfer skillet to oven and cook 40 minutes or until vegetables are tender. Serve with a roast chicken (p. 222).

Root vegetables en chemise

Cooked in parchment packets, vegetables will retain all of their flavors and all of their nutritional properties.

Ingredients (4 servings)

2 tsp olive oil
2 tbsp lemon juice
Zest of 1 lemon, grated
1 clove of garlic, minced
2 tsp salted herbs
2 carrots, julienned (about 2 inches long)
2 parsnip, julienned (about 2 inches long)
1 small turnip, julienned (about 2 inches long)
1 long sheet of parchment paper

✿ Parsnip

Rich in mineral salts and insoluble fiber, parsnip is the perfect vegetable for anyone wanting to lose weight. Its delicate and subtle taste add personality to soups, stews and mashed vegetables.

Preparation

▮ Preheat oven to 400°F.
▮ In a salad bowl, mix together oil, lemon juice and zest, salted herbs and garlic.
▮ Add vegetables and mix well with your hands to coat thoroughly with marinade.
▮ Lay vegetables on parchment paper and fold over to make a large packet; place on baking sheet.
▮ Cook in the oven for 45 minutes or until vegetables are tender.

Note

▮ If you want to serve these vegetables with a roast, cook at the same time as the meat, but at a lower temperature. They will need to cook a little longer. In a 350°F oven, cook for 1 ¼ hours; in a 350°F oven, cook for 1 hour.

Herb and garlic potatoes

Garlic lovers, get your tastebuds ready! It's time to honor the piquant little bulb.

Ingredients (4 servings)

16 small, baby potatoes, quartered

3 tbsp olive oil

2 tsp fresh garlic, chopped

2 tsp fresh rosemary or thyme, or any other dried or fresh herb

Salt and pepper to taste

Preparation

▌ Preheat oven to 325°F.

▌ In a shallow baking dish, combine potatoes, oil, garlic and herbs.

▌ Cook uncovered 1 hour or until potatoes are tender.

▌ Add salt and pepper before serving.

Cherry nutty quinoa

An ancient grain, quinoa has just recently found its way to our pantries. It is one of the few cereals to contain all eight essential amino-acids. Spiced up and flavored with orange, it is absolutely delicious.

Ingredients (4 servings)

1 cup quinoa, thoroughly rinsed and drained

2 cups water

½ tsp salt

1 tsp dried basil

1 tsp cajun mix (p. 253)

¼ tsp cinnamon

1 tsp orange zest, grated

⅓ cup dried cherries

¼ cup cashews, toasted and coarsely chopped

Preparation

▌ Cook quinoa in boiling salt water, following instructions on package. Usually, it needs to simmer 10 minutes uncovered until grains become translucent; then remove from heat, cover and let swell 5 minutes.

▌ Season with basil, cajun mix, cinnamon and orange zest; then incorporate cherries and nuts.

▌ Taste, adjust seasoning and serve warm or cold.

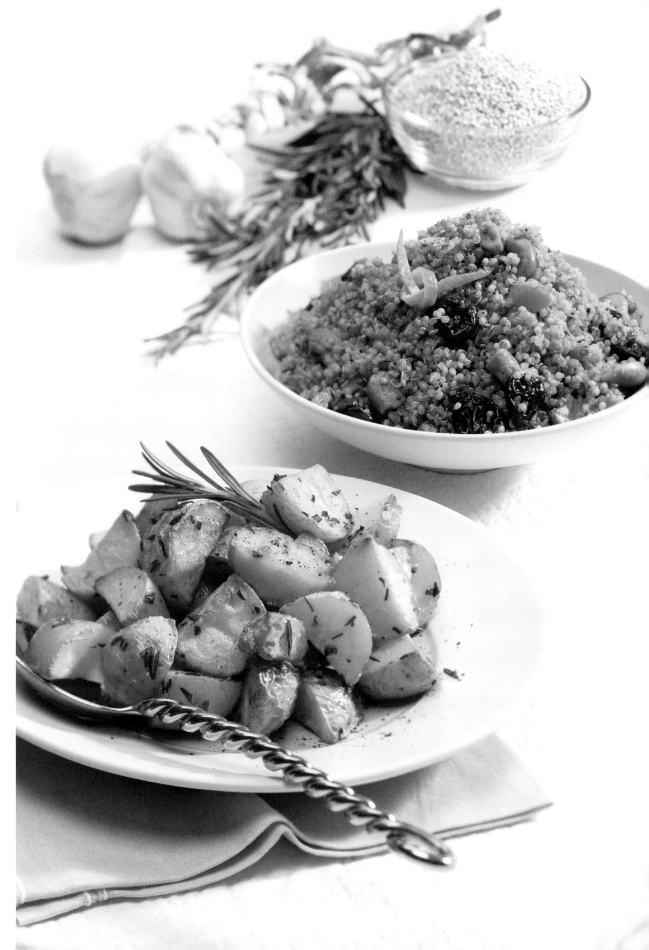

Mashed parsnip, carrot and sweet potato

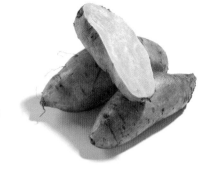

This purée is delicious with duck or rabbit. It can be prepared ahead of time and reheated in the microwave just before serving.

Ingredients (4 servings)

2 parsnips, peeled and cut in pieces
3 medium carrots, peeled and cut in pieces
1 large sweet potato, peeled and cut in pieces
Salt water
1 tbsp non-hydrogenated margarine
Pinch of nutmeg
½ tsp cajun spice mix (p. 253)
½ tsp turmeric
2 tbsp fresh parsley, chopped

Preparation

▌ In a pot of salt water, bring parsnip, carrot and sweet potato to a boil. Lower heat and simmer 15 minutes or until vegetables are tender. Drain thoroughly.
▌ Mash vegetables with an electric mixer.
▌ Melt margarine in the microwave for 30 seconds, add nutmeg and spices; pour on purée. Add parsley and stir well to mix.
▌ Serve hot.

Sweet potato and apple purée

A nice delicate side dish to accompany roasted poultry, this purée is infused with the fragrances of turmeric and orange.

Ingredients (4 servings)

1 sweet potato, peeled and cut in cubes
   (about 4 cups)
1 tbsp non-hydrogenated margarine
1 cooking apple, peeled and grated
1 dry shallot, minced
¼ tsp nutmeg
¼ tsp chili flakes
½ tsp turmeric
1 tsp orange zest, grated
¼ cup fresh parsley, chopped
Salt and pepper to taste

Preparation

▌ In a pot of cold salt water, put sweet potato pieces, cover and bring to a boil. Lower heat and simmer 15 minutes.
▌ In a small frying pan, melt margarine and sauté grated apple and shallot for 5 minutes.
▌ Purée sweet potato, incorporate apple, nutmeg, chili flakes, turmeric, orange zest and parsley.
▌ Serve with chicken or duck.

Rice infused with apple and orange

Turmeric and chili pepper delicately flavor this microwave-cooked rice, giving it a little kick. Delicious served with roast chicken or grilled fish.

Ingredients (4 servings or more)

2 tbsp oil
1 dry shallot, minced
1 cup long grain white rice
¾ cup apple juice
1 ½ cups chicken broth (p. 145)
1 tsp turmeric
½ tsp hot sauce
Salt and pepper to taste
3 tbsp unsweetened coconut flakes
1 tsp orange zest
½ cup pistachios
Salt and pepper to taste

Preparation

▌ In a large microwave-safe measuring cup, combine oil and shallot; microwave on high for 1 minute.

▌ Add rice, mixing to coat well with oil and shallot; microwave on high for 1 minute.

▌ Add apple juice, broth, turmeric, hot sauce, coconut flakes, salt and pepper; cover loosely with plastic wrap and microwave on high for 8 minutes. Continue cooking on medium power for 10 minutes or until liquid is almost absorbed.

▌ If a lot of liquid remains, microwave on high for 1 or 2 more minutes.

▌ Incorporate orange zest and pistachios, let rest about 5 minutes before serving.

Spicy sweet pepper rice

Sweet peppers and hot sauce infuse this microwave rice with their antioxidant and anti-inflammatory powers, which are so valuable to arthritis sufferers.

Ingredients (4 servings)

2 tbsp olive oil
1 leek (whites), minced or 2 dry shallots, minced
Half a sweet red pepper, diced
Half a sweet yellow pepper, diced
½ tsp celery seeds, ground
½ tsp hot sauce
1 cup long grain rice
2 cups water with ¾ tsp salt

Preparation

▌ In a large 8-cup microwave-safe bowl or measuring cup, combine oil, leek whites and sweet pepper.

▌ Microwave on high for 1 minutes.

▌ Add rice, celery seeds and hot sauce; mix and cook for 1 minute.

▌ Add salt water and microwave on high for 8 minutes.

▌ Continue cooking at medium power for 10 more minutes.

▌ Let rest 5 minutes before serving.

Sauces, vinaigrettes and dips

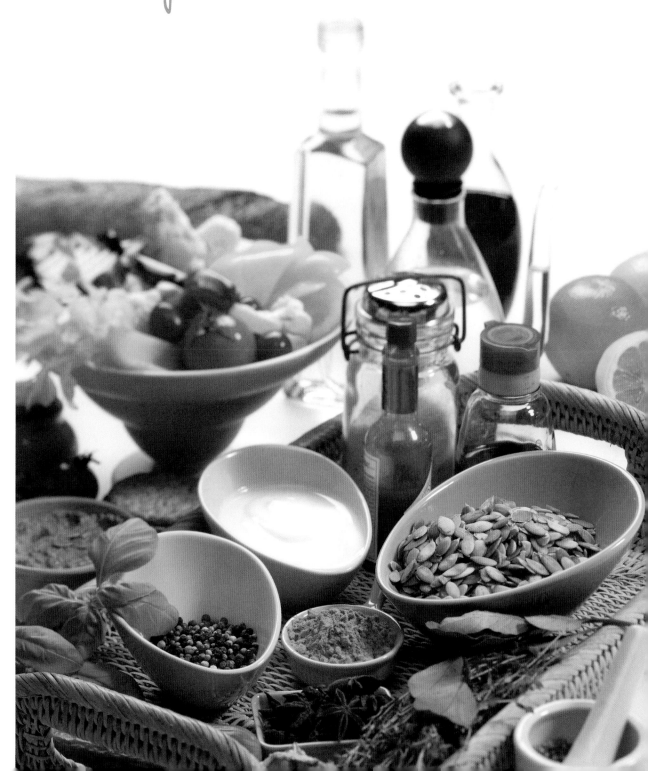

Taste enhancers

Sauces, vinaigrettes and dips are against monotony and routine; they are agents of flavor. As the secret to a good soup is very often the quality of its broth, the hidden flavors in a salad are revealed by the dressing that... dresses it up! The flavor of a dish with two or three vegetables will really pop with a splash of lemon and tarragon vinaigrette, or with a smattering of cilantro pesto. Furthermore, a rich tomato sauce or tangy pesto dressing can transform an ordinary pasta or bean dish from ho-hum to simply yum!

Sauces, vinaigrettes and dips

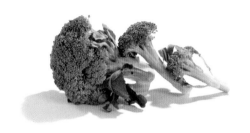

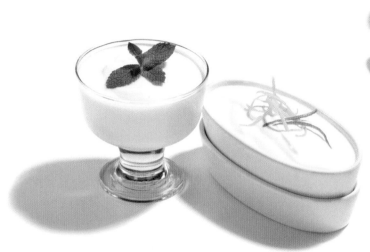

Wheat germ oil vinaigrette

This bold tasting vinaigrette is perfect for salads made with cabbage, celery or sweet peppers.

Ingredients (4 servings)

1 tbsp cider vinegar
1 tsp Dijon mustard
Pinch of salted herbs
Pinch of cayenne pepper
3 tbsp olive oil
1 tbsp wheat germ oil
Pepper to taste

Preparation

- In a small bowl, mix together vinegar, mustard, salted herbs and cayenne pepper.
- Add salt and pepper, slowly incorporate the two oils and emulsify.

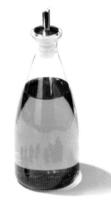

Orange and curry vinaigrette

This vinaigrette is delicious with a fresh fruit salad of mango, papaya, pineapple, pear, and/or strawberry on their own or in any combination together.

Ingredients (6-8 servings)

1 tsp Dijon mustard
2 tsp orange zest, grated
1 tsp curry powder
1 tsp turmeric
½ tsp fresh ginger, minced
¼ tsp cumin
½ cup fresh orange juice
3 tbsp olive oil

Preparation

- In a small bowl, whisk together all the ingredients. Refrigerate 1 hour for the flavors to develop and mingle.

 Curry

Curry powder is a blend of spices called "garam masala" in India. It is a combination of fragrant aromatics: cloves, coriander, cumin, turmeric, cardamom, fenugreek and cayenne pepper. Ground with a mortar and pestle, then heated in a skillet, theses spices will infuse any dish from soups to desserts with their exotic perfume.

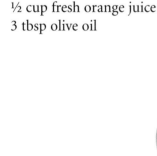

Lemon and tarragon vinaigrette

Drizzle this vinaigrette on al dente asparagus, steamed snow peas, or broccoli and cauliflower florets.

Ingredients (4 servings)

1 tsp lemon juice
1 tsp lemon zest, grated
1 small clove of garlic, minced
1 tbsp cider vinegar
½ tsp honey
4 tbsp olive oil
2 tsp fresh tarragon or 1 tsp dried tarragon
Salt and pepper to taste

Preparation

▌ In a small bowl, combine lemon juice, lemon zest and garlic.
▌ Incorporate vinegar and honey, then olive oil, tarragon, salt and pepper and mix well.

Firm yogurt with dried herbs

This super easy and delicately fragrant yogurt dip is inspired by Middle Eastern cuisine.

Ingredients (1 cup)

1 cup plain yogurt
1 tsp dried herbs (basil, mint, oregano)
1 tbsp fresh parsley, chopped
Salt and pepper to taste
Piece of cheesecloth or coffee filter

Preparation

▌ Combine yogurt with herbs and parsley, season with salt and pepper. Put yogurt mixture in a strainer lined with cheesecloth or coffee filter and place over a bowl. Cover and refrigerate for 24 hours.

✿ Yogurt

Yogurt is a very healthy food as long as it is unsweetened and has no additives. It contains calcium, phosphorus, and potassium as well as vitamins A and B. The bacteria in yogurt can prevent mycotic infections, and stimulate good bacteria and kill harmful bacteria in the body.

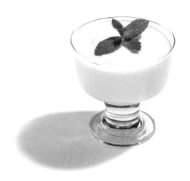

Pumpkin seed dip

Dips enhance the taste of all vegetables, including those beneficial to arthritis sufferers. Many different kinds of seeds contain nutrients that lend therapeutic properties to the foods they are prepared with, such as sauces and dips. Easy, fast and delicious!

Ingredients

¼ cup pumpkin seeds, ground
1 small dry shallot, chopped
¼ cup fresh parsley leaves, chopped
¼ tsp chili flakes
1 small tomato, seeded and chopped
1 tbsp plain yogurt
Salt and pepper to taste

Preparation

▌ In a blender or food processor, combine ground pumpkin seeds, dry shallot, parsley and chili flakes; process until coarsely puréed. Add tomatoes and process again until smooth in consistency.

▌ Incorporate yogurt, mix well and refrigerate 30 minutes. Serve with crudités and on crackers.

Sun-dried tomato dip

This flavorful dip goes well with crudités, but can also be added to soups or sprinkled with cheese and spread on crackers.

Ingredients

¼ cup dried tomatoes (not packed in oil), very finely chopped
¼ cup plain yogurt
¼ tsp dried oregano
¼ tsp dried thyme
2 tbsp fresh parsley, chopped
Dash of hot sauce
Salt and pepper

Preparation

▌ If dried tomatoes are too tough, soak for 30 minutes in ½ cup boiling water. Rinse and drain, then mix thoroughly with yogurt, mashing them to blend well. Add herbs, spices and seasonings. Add more yogurt if necessary to adjust consistency. Serve with crudités.

Gourmet touch

▌ Add 2 tbsp parmesan.

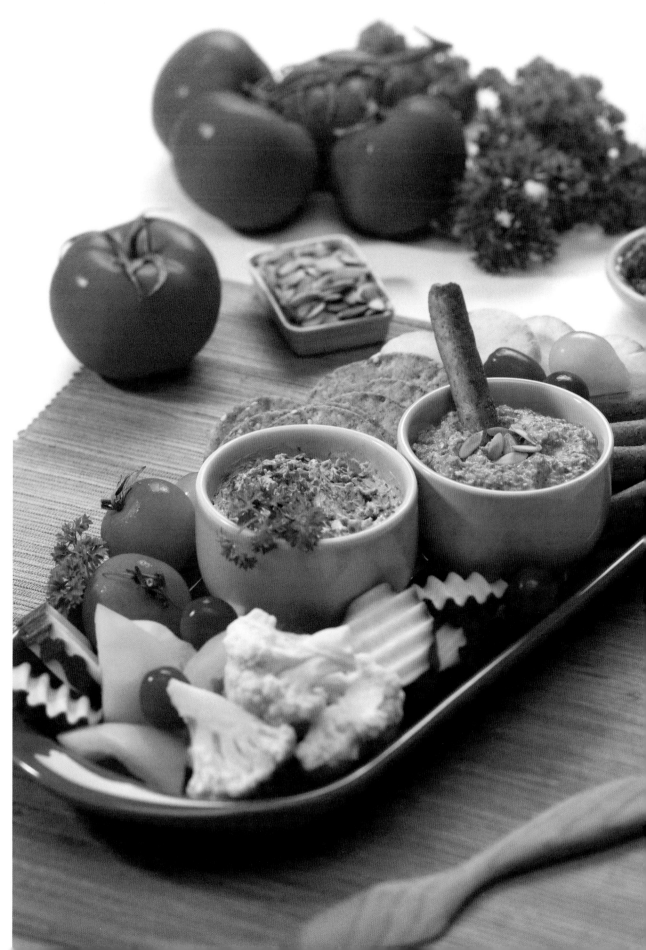

Pizza sauce

This tomato sauce is easy to make and versatile. It's delicious on pasta, fish, beans or chicken. You will want to have some on hand at all times, so double up the recipe to freeze in portioned containers.

Ingredients (2 cups)

18 ounce can whole tomatoes
2 tbsp tomato paste
1 small onion, chopped
2 cloves of garlic, minced
½ tsp basil
½ tsp oregano
¼ tsp chili flakes
Salt and pepper to taste

Preparation

▌ In a blender or food processor, purée all of the ingredients until desired consistency.

▌ Pour mixture in a saucepan and bring to a boil. Lower heat and simmer uncovered for 30 minutes until sauce thickens, stirring occasionally.

▌ Add salt and pepper and cool. Use immediately or freeze in portioned containers.

Basic tomato sauce

As with most traditional Italian dishes, this sauce requires few ingredients and is simply delicious. Double the recipe and freeze in portioned containers to have on hand for whenever culinary inspiration strikes.

Ingredients (6 servings)

4 tbsp olive oil
4 cloves of garlic, minced
2 cans (18 ounces each) plum tomatoes, puréed
  with a hand mixer*
3 tbsp olive oil
Salt and pepper to taste

* *This gives the sauce a rich, smooth texture.*

Preparation

▌ In a saucepan, heat some oil and gently cook garlic 5 minutes or so without letting it color.

▌ Add tomato, the 3 tbsp of olive oil and partially cover to thicken sauce. Bring to a boil, lower heat and simmer gently for 1 hour.

▌ Remove from heat before adding salt and pepper.

Picante variation

▌ For a spicier sauce, add ½ or 1 teaspoon of chili flakes.

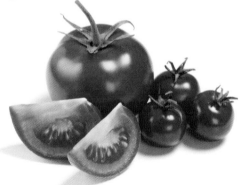

Cilantro pesto

Ingredients (½ cup)

¼ cup unsalted hazelnuts
1 cup fresh cilantro, chopped
1 cup fresh parsley, chopped
3 cloves of garlic, minced
2 tbsp chicken broth (p. 145)
¼ cup canola oil
Salt and pepper to taste

Preparation

▌ In a blender or food processor, chop hazelnuts and set aside.

▌ In a blender or food processor, combine chopped cilantro and parsley, garlic and chicken broth. Process.

▌ Add oil and purée until smooth. Add chopped hazelnuts, season to taste and mix again until desired consistency.

Basil and pistachio pesto

Ingredients (¼ cup)

1 clove of garlic, minced
2 tbsp pistachios, chopped
½ cup fresh parsley, chopped
½ cup fresh basil leaves, chopped
2 tbsp chicken broth (p. 145)
4 tbsp canola or olive oil
Salt and pepper to taste

Preparation

▌ In a blender or food processor, chop pistachios. Add garlic, parsley, basil and broth; purée. Slowly pour in oil as the mixture is being processed until a smooth consistency is reached. Add salt and pepper, serve.

Quick winter pesto

Ingredients (½ cup)

½ cup pecans
1 cup fresh parsley, rinsed and chopped
1 tsp dried basil
2 cloves of garlic, minced
¼ cup olive oil
2 2 tbsp chicken broth (p. 145) or more if needed
Salt and pepper to taste

Preparation

▌ Preheat oven to 350°F.

▌ Toast pecans 5 minutes in the oven until golden and fragrant.

▌ In a blender or food processor, coarsely chop pecans and remove.

▌ In blender or food processor, combine parsley, basil, garlic and oil. Pulse, incorporate pecans, mix well and season. If mixture is too thick, add broth one spoonful at a time until desired consistency is achieved.

Spice mixes

Make your own spice blends to give a variety of flavors to the dishes you cook. All you need to do is grind different seeds with a mortar and pestle or in a coffee grinder (you might want to reserve it for spice-grinding only as it might make for a spicy-tasting cup of coffee!) Once you have ground and measured your spices, keep them in closed glass containers, labeled and kept in a dark, dry place. The flavors will continue to develop and will reach their peak in the first weeks of storage. That is why it is best to prepare only small quantities at a time.

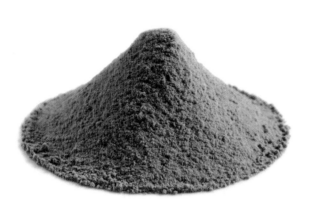

Indian spice mix

Ingredients

1 tsp cumin, ground
1 tsp coriander, ground
½ tsp fenugreek
1 tsp turmeric
¼ tsp cardamom, ground
½ tsp cayenne pepper

Preparation

▮ Grind herbs and spices as needed and mix. Store in a glass container away from light.

Chili seasoning

Ingredients

½ tsp black pepper
½ tsp ground clove
1 tsp cumin, ground
1 tsp cayenne pepper
2 tsp oregano, ground
4 tsp paprika

Preparation

▌ Grind herbs and spices as needed and mix.
Store in a glass container away from light.

Cajun spice mix

Ingredients

1 tsp chili flakes, crushed
3 tsp paprika
1 tsp oregano, ground
1 tsp thyme, ground
1 tsp black pepper, ground

Preparation

▌ Grind herbs and spices as needed and mix.
Store in a glass container away from light.

Maghrebian spice mix

Ingredients

1 tsp cumin
1 tsp coriander
1 tsp fennel seeds, ground
1 tsp dried basil
1 tsp dried mint
¼ tsp chili flakes, crushed

Preparation

▌ Grind herbs and spices as needed and mix.
Store in a glass container away from light.

Moroccan spice mix

Ingredients

2 tsp cumin, ground
2 tsp coriander, ground
2 tsp ginger, ground
1 tsp chili seasoning
½ tsp black pepper
½ tsp turmeric
½ tsp cinnamon, ground
½ tsp salt
¼ tsp ground clove

Preparation

▌ Grind herbs and spices as needed and mix.
Store in a glass container away from light.

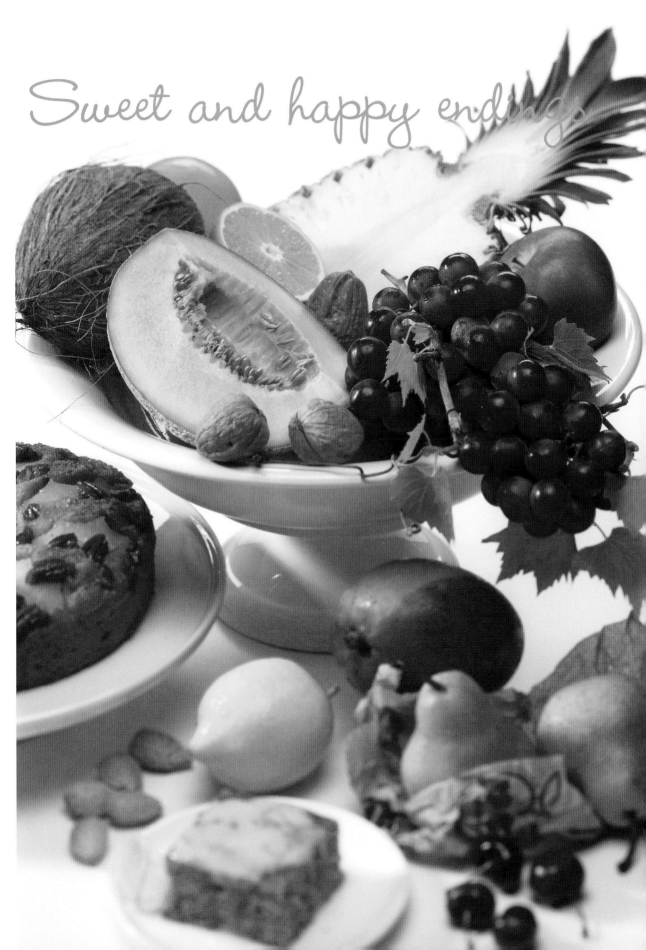

Sweet and happy endings

Fruity desserts

The grand finale to a great meal should be sweet, but not too heavy. These easy-to-make desserts are filled with healthy, delicious fruit.

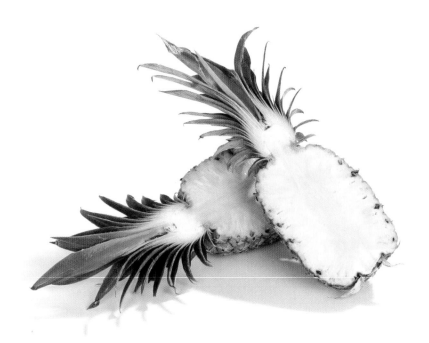

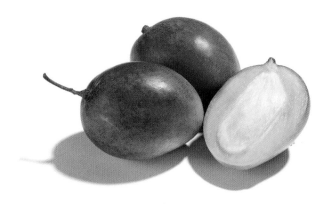

Sweet and happy endings

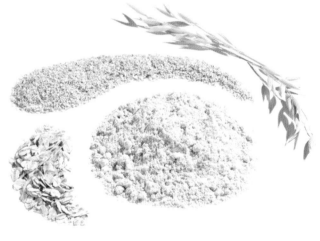

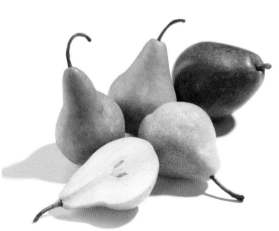

Yogurt and poppy seeds squares

This light cake draped with a tangy yogurt and lemon sauce, is the perfect way to end a summer feast.

Ingredients (6 servings)

1 egg
½ cup sugar
1 tsp almond extract
1 tsp orange zest
⅓ cup canola oil
1 cup whole wheat pastry flour
1 tsp baking powder
¼ cup strained yogurt*
¼ cup vanilla soy milk
⅓ cup poppy seeds
1 tsp non-hydrogenated margarine

* *Straining yogurt for a few hours or overnight gives it a firm, smooth texture. Put it in the fridge in a cheesecloth-lined strainer placed over a bowl and covered with plastic wrap.*

Preparation

▋ Preheat oven to 325°F.
▋ In a bowl, beat egg with sugar, almond extract and orange zest on high speed for two minutes. Add oil and beat 30 seconds at low speed.
▋ In another bowl, combine flour and baking powder.
▋ Add dry ingredients to the egg mixture alternating with yogurt and soy milk at low speed, being careful not to overmix.
▋ Incorporate poppy seeds by folding them in with a spatula.
▋ Spread batter in an 8-inch square pan brushed with margarine and bake 1 hour.
▋ Allow to cool and enjoy plain or topped with lemon icing or a fruit compote.

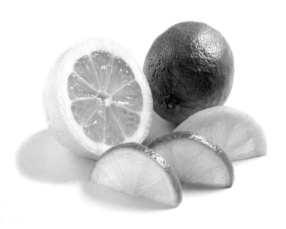

Lemon icing

½ cup icing sugar
¼ cup plain yogurt
½ tsp lemon zest
½ tsp lemon juice

Preparation

▋ In a small bowl, combine all ingredients.
▋ Mix well and spoon on cake.

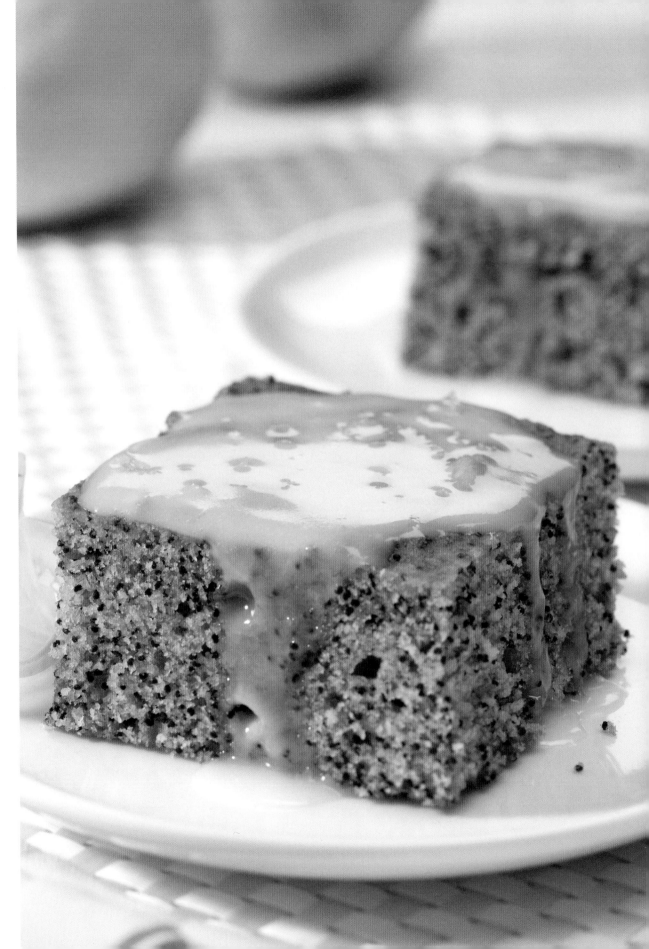

Frosty clementines

This is a quick and easy dessert, perfect to make with the kids.

Ingredients (4 servings)

4 unpeeled clementines
⅔ cup frozen vanilla yogurt
4 cherries or hazelnuts and some mint leaves
  to garnish

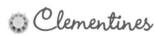 **Clementines**

Kids love this tiny, juicy fruit loaded with
vitamin C and flavonoids. It comes in very
handy when only a small quantity of orange
juice is needed for a recipe.

Preparation

▮ Cut a quarter-sized hole in each clementine,
  using a paring knife. Spoon out flesh through
  the opening. Save the juice for other uses, to
  make a vinaigrette for example. Chop the
  flesh, mix it with yogurt and fill the hollowed
  clementines with this mixture.

▮ Freeze 1 hour before placing in pretty dessert
  cups. Garnish with cherries or hazelnuts, surround with mint leaves.

Mango cream express

Don't be deceived by how simple this recipe appears; it is absolutely delicious.

Ingredients (4 servings)

2 ripe mangos, peeled and cut in pieces
4 tbsp coconut milk
Mint leaves for garnish

Preparation

▮ In a blender or food processor, combine
  mango pieces and coconut milk. Purée until
  consistency is smooth and creamy; pour in
  pretty dessert cups. Garnish with mint leaves
  and serve.

Tip

▮ Don't forget that you can freeze leftover coconut milk.

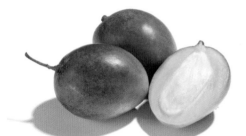

Crispy rice and date bites

Another quick and easy dessert that also makes a great snack.

Ingredients – (about 24 bite-size balls)

1 cup dates, pitted and chopped
¼ cup non-hydrogenated margarine
¼ cup brown sugar
1 tbsp lemon juice
½ cup shredded coconut
2 cups crispy rice cereal (like Rice Crispies)
½ cup unsalted sunflower seeds

Preparation

▌ In a saucepan, combine dates, margarine, brown sugar and lemon juice. Cook 5 minutes over medium heat stirring constantly until mixture becomes syrupy. Remove from heat and pour in a bowl.

▌ Incorporate cococut, rice cereal and sunflower seeds. Shape bite-size balls, spread out on a baking sheet and cool 30 minutes in the fridge.

▌ Store any leftovers in an airtight container in the fridge.

Pear rice pudding

This easy dessert is a good way to use up leftover rice; it doesn't matter if it is a little salty.

Ingredients (4 servings)

1 cup cooked rice
2 tbsp brown sugar
2 tbsp coconut flakes
1 egg, beaten
½ cup vanilla soy milk
½ tsp almond extract
3 pears, peeled and cut in pieces

Preparation

▌ Preheat oven to 350°F.

▌ In a bowl, combine all the ingredients except for the pear and mix well with a fork.

▌ Pour in a Pyrex baking dish, add pear pieces pushing them into the mixture. Bake for 40 minutes.

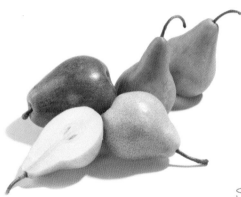

Pineapple upside down cake

This classic dessert is always a hit with its crown of fruit garnished with pecans.

Ingredients (8 servings)

Topping
3 pineapple slices, cut in three
¼ cup non-hydrogenated margarine
½ cup brown sugar
¼ cup pecans, coarsely chopped

Cake
½ cup non-hydrogenated margarine
1 tsp vanilla extract
½ cup brown sugar
2 large eggs
1 ½ cups pastry flour
1 ½ tsp baking powder
Pinch of salt
½ cup plain soy milk

Preparation

▌ Preheat oven to 350°F.
▌ In a small bowl, combine margarine and brown sugar.
▌ In an 8-inch tube pan (Bundt pan) coated with margarine, spread batter and sprinkle with pecan and pineapple pieces.
▌ In another bowl, using an electric mixer, beat margarine, vanilla extract and brown sugar. Add eggs one at a time, beating well after each one.
▌ Incorporate dry sifted ingredients to this mixture alternating with soy milk while beating with a wooden spoon. Spread over pineapple.
▌ Bake 40 minutes or until a toothpick inserted in the centre comes out clean.
▌ Let rest 5 minutes before turning over onto a plate. Serve warm or cold.

❀ Pineapple

Pineapple contains vitamin C and beta-carotein but its high content of bromelin (an enzyme that breaks down protein) is what makes it particularly helpful to relieve joint pain.

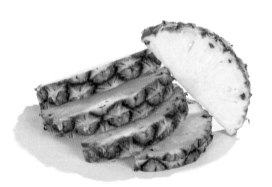

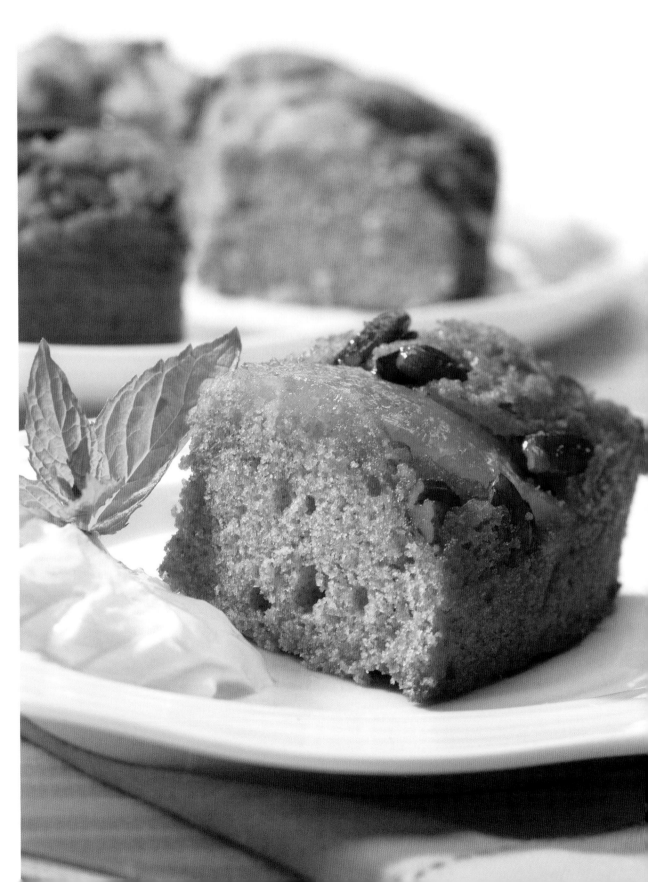

Quick rolled oat cookies

Perfect to pack in a lunch box or to enjoy alongside a fruit salad, these healthy cookies take no time to make, and even less time to disappear.

Ingredients (24 cookies)

½ cup non-hydrogenated margarine
½ cup packed brown sugar
1 egg, beaten
1 cup whole wheat pastry flour
1 cup quick-cook rolled oats
¼ cup wheat germ
1 tsp baking powder
1 tsp baking soda
½ tsp each of the following ground spices:
    cinnamon, clove, ginger
1 cup sunflower seeds
2 tbsp olive oil

 Oats

Oat is a cereal known for its stabilizing effect on blood sugar and is therefore beneficial to diabetics. Get into the habit of mixing rolled oats in with your bread crumbs to enrich any foods you would usually bread, like meat croquettes. And don't forget to add it to desserts!

Preparation

▌ Preheat oven to 350°F.

▌ In a bowl, cream margarine and brown sugar together until fluffly.

▌ In another bowl, combine dry ingredients: flour, oats, wheat germ, baking powder, baking soda and spices; mix well.

▌ Add dry mixture to margarine mixture gradually alternating with beaten egg. Incorporate sunflower seeds.

▌ If mixture is dry and crumbly, add 1 or 2 tbsp of olive oil.

▌ Separate dough in two large balls; form 12 smaller balls, the size of walnuts, with each half.

▌ On a baking sheet lightly brushed with margarine, place 12 balls of dough, flattening to make 12 cookies 2 inches in diameter.

▌ Bake 10 to 12 minutes.

▌ Place cookies on a wire rack with a spatula to cool.

▌ Repeat with the 12 remaining dough balls.

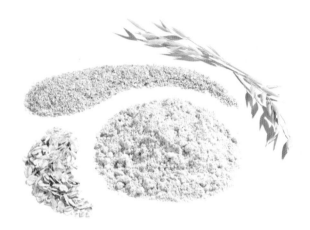

Carrot cake

This cake is so delicious, it doesn't need any frosting. It is a sheer delight served with a clementine and turmeric sauce (p. 130).

Ingredients (4 to 6 servings)

½ cup brown sugar
4 tbsp canola oil
½ cup apple juice
2 large eggs, slightly beaten
1 ⅔ cups pastry flour
2 tsp baking powder
1 tsp orange zest, grated
2 cups finely grated carrot (about 2 large carrots)

Preparation

▌ Preheat oven to 325°F.
▌ In a large bowl, mix brown sugar and oil. Add apple juice and eggs.
▌ In another bowl, mix flour with baking powder. Incorporate dry ingredients gradually with wet ingredients, beating well. Add carrots and beat until batter is smooth.
▌ Pour in an 8-inch square baking pan brushed with margarine.
▌ Bake 50 minutes or until a toothpick inserted in the center comes out clean.
▌ Cool in the pan 10 minutes before turning out onto a rack.

Curried fruit salad

Fresh fruit macerating in a fragrant sauce of orange and curry is a delicious way to end a meal.

Ingredients (4 servings)

2 ½ cups fresh fruit cut in bite-size pieces (mango, cantaloupe, pineapple)
½ cup red grapes, halved

Curry sauce
1 tsp orange zest, grated
½ tsp curry powder
½ tsp turmeric
½ tsp fresh ginger, finely grated
½ tsp vanilla extract
1 tsp honey
½ cup fresh orange juice

Preparation

▌ In a salad bowl, combine all fruit.
▌ In a small bowl, whisk together all the sauce ingredients.
▌ Pour onto fruit and refrigerate 3 hours to let the flavors develop.
▌ Add the grape halves and serve on its own or with frozen yogurt.

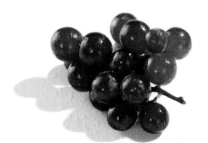

Ginger apple crisp

Ginger marmalade gives this delicious dessert a nice zing.

Ingredients (4 servings)

4 cups apple, peeled and cubed
5 tbsp ginger marmalade
Juice and grated zest of one orange
½ cup rolled oats or unsweetened cereal flakes, crushed
½ cup pastry flour
¼ cup packed brown sugar
¼ cup pecans, coarsely chopped
5 tbsp non-hydrogenated margarine

Preparation

▌ Preheat oven to 375°F.
▌ In a bowl, combine apple, marmalade, orange juice and zest; mix well. Spread mixture in a 9-inch square pan brushed with margarine.
▌ In another bowl, combine rolled oats or cereal, flour, brown sugar and nuts; mix well. Add margarine and mix until consistency resembles bread crumbs. Spread this mixture over the apples.
▌ Bake 35 to 45 minutes until the apples are tender. Serve warm.

Pear variation

▌ Substitute the pear for apple, the ginger marmalade for orange marmalade, and omit the orange zest for a tasty pear crisp.

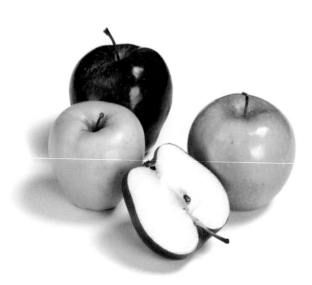

Recipe Index

General Index

These terms can be found in Part One and Part Two, as well as in the introduction to Part Three. Sections dedicated to a particular food are indicated in bold. Each section includes a list of recipes featuring the healing food and provides page numbers for the recipes.

Table of contents

Part Three – Cooking for pleasure